Motility in Osteopathy

From embryology to clinical practice

Motility in Osteopathy

From embryology to clinical practice

Alain Auberville, diplômée en ostéopathie,
Osteopathy practitioner,
Co-founder of l'Institut Supérieur d'ostéopathie,
(Aix-en-Provence, France)

Andrée Aubin, diplômée en ostéopathie,
Osteopathy practitioner,
Director and Teacher, Centre Ostéopathique
du Québec (Montréal, Canada)

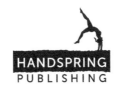

HANDSPRING
PUBLISHING

EDINBURGH

HANDSPRING PUBLISHING LIMITED
The Old Manse, Fountainhall,
Pencaitland, East Lothian
EH34 5EY, Scotland
Tel: +44 1875 341 859
Website: www.handspringpublishing.com

Originally published in 2015 in French by Elsevier Masson
First published in 2017 in English by Handspring Publishing

© 2015, Elsevier Masson. Tous droits réservés

This edition of **La motilité en ostéopathie. Nouveau concept basé sur l'embryologie** by **Alain Auberville & Andrée Aubin** is published by arrangement with Elsevier Masson SAS.

Copyright © Handspring Publishing 2017
Illustrations by Renée Othot

ISBN 978-1-909141-66-7

British Library Cataloguing in Publication Data
A catalogue record for this book is available from the British Library

Library of Congress Cataloguing in Publication Data
A catalog record for this book is available from the Library of Congress

Notice
Neither the Publisher nor the Author assumes any responsibility for any loss or injury and/or damage to persons or property arising out of or relating to any use of the material contained in this book. It is the responsibility of the treating practitioner, relying on independent expertise and knowledge of the patient, to determine the best treatment and method of application for the patient.

Commissioning Editor Mary Law
Project Manager Morven Dean
Translator Louis Goulet
Copy Editor Sally Davies
Typesetter DSMSoft
Printer Ashford Colour Press Ltd

The
Publisher's
policy is to use
paper manufactured
from sustainable forests

Contents

The authors

Alain Auberville

After practicing as a physiotherapist from 1965 to 1983, Alain Auberville qualified as an osteopath in 1984. He then went on to complete his professional development by studying naturopathy and Chinese medicine. He was involved in founding the osteopathy schools Eurostéo and InSO-Aix-en-Provence, where he taught the visceral approach to osteopathy. He now practices at Pélissanne, in the south of France.

Dr Auberville has developed his embryology-based motility concept over the last 30 years by experimenting and clinically validating his hypothesis. He has extended the concept for all the structures and the visceral, neurological and musculoskeletal systems of the body. He has been teaching this concept and its applications for more than 15 years to students of the schools he co-founded in France as well as to those attending courses at the Centre Ostéopathique du Québec, Canada.

He teaches postgraduate courses, notably in France, Italy, and Russia.

Andrée Aubin

Andrée Aubin graduated in physiotherapy at the University of Montreal in 1986. She has run a private osteopathy practice since 1992 when she obtained her osteopathy degree at the Centre Ostéopathique du Québec (COQ, Montreal). She is currently general manager of the Centre Ostéopathique du Québec where she has also been teaching for over 23 years. Her expertise concerns the cranial field, osteopathic teaching methods (especially for palpation skills), management of complex cases and the clinical reasoning process. In recent years, she has contributed to several OsEAN Open Forums. Since 2013, she has been involved in the creation of an osteopathic Master's degree program at the University of Sherbrooke. She occasionally offers postgraduate courses outside Canada, in France and Spain.

It was in 1984–1985 that, newly qualified in osteopathy and studying at the Société Française d'Enseignement et de Recherche en Énergétique (SFERE), I first came across the osteopath and teacher Alain Ripert, who shared with us his ideas on possible relationships between Chinese traditional medicine and embryology, based on chronology and vital energy flow.

Chinese traditional medicine is based on this flow of energy, its movement, and osteopathy's foundation is also movement. During embryogenesis, nearly all of the embryo's structures will move, carried by energy! With these ideas in mind, I wished to find new osteopathic techniques that would make use of the principles of Chinese medicine in my clinical practice. Embryology suits this purpose by combining movement and energy.

I started by looking into embryogenesis and, more precisely, its associated movements, such as the migrations and proliferation of the cells that ultimately make up all the structures of the body, following an unalterable chronology.

The first tests and techniques that I developed based on embryology development were for the digestive system. They have been used on thousands of patients in different clinical contexts, particularly when traditional osteopathic techniques did not deliver the desired results. This intensive use made me realize it was often possible to normalize dysfunctions in a quicker and more efficient way by using these motility techniques. Furthermore, mobility dysfunctions often disappeared following just the motility treatment, implying they were adaptive and not necessarily independent, and that motility could be, in many cases, preferred over mobility.

SFERE had a device to measure electrical potential differences at the acupuncture points, so we were able to verify the positive results of the motility treatment in an objective way, which persuaded me to commit to this approach.

Visceral osteopathy, as taught at SFERE and also in osteopathy schools across Europe and North America, made the development of this concept possible and even helped shape and define it, thanks to the students' insight and questions.

The embryology-based motility concept then expanded to encompass the urogenital and cardiopulmonary systems, with equally interesting results.

At that time, I questioned the variable results of classical diaphragm treatment techniques. Why did some diaphragm dysfunctions react quickly to spheno-occipital synostosis decompression techniques – so quickly that it might imply a neurological action on the pneumotaxic center – when others did not react at all? How could we intervene directly on the superior centers? Were they responsible for the persistence of some of these dysfunctions?

In the late 1980s, these questions led me to apply the energetic motility concept to the autonomic and central nervous systems. Important embryological movements in the midbrain and pontine flexures were my first concern. Working on the neurological field broadened my osteopathic practice, leading to new reasons for consultation and better results for many of the existing reasons for consultation.

To my great satisfaction, these 'neuro' techniques enabled me to lift dysfunctions causing reflex algoneurodystrophy, a painful and disabling condition for which too few effective therapeutic resources exist. The patients who were treated and also I myself were surprised by how effective the treatment of neurological motility losses was and how quickly the patients recovered. Some of them even experienced the remineralization of bones as a consequence of the treatment, which made me realize that the line between structure and function is certainly thinner than their definitions imply. At this time the possibilities for osteopathy expanded for me.

Some long-standing questions about the sacrum remained unanswered: why did its felt movement seem to be much more extensive than its theoretical counterpart, which is supposed to be only a mirror of cranial movement? How to explain the mechanical contradiction in the osteopathic explanation of whiplash? The study of the third and fourth weeks of embryological development, in which the caudal part of the body undergoes a lot of movement – movement named, in this work, caudal plication – gave me some answers. If the fold formed by the unrolling of the inferior part of the embryo was perceivable, and understanding it was able to lead to new treatments, why wouldn't it be the same with the superior part of the body's movements, such as the one that leads the heart to its place in the thorax? This is how, in the early 1980s, the idea of thoracic and caudal plication came to life, and was later refined by clinical experimentation and theoretical analysis.

Working on energy progressively made its way into both my mind and my practice, forming a coherent system the implementation of which followed a clear protocol and chronology based on the steps of human development and on the neurological pathways maintaining physical health. This system might seem to be far from traditional osteopathy at first; however, it follows the basic concept of osteopathic movement and its underlying principles, requiring only a questioning and deepening of knowledge to extend their essence.

The direction of this work evolved through clinical experimentation, discussions with a few enthusiastic colleagues, and mostly thanks to the positive feedback given by successfully treated patients. Some of these cases will be covered briefly in Chapter 10, and illustrate the various potential effects of the proposed techniques. I am thankful to my patients, who taught me so much; their continued trust is my most treasured reward.

I hope you take as much pleasure in the study of this work as I did.

Alain Auberville, Pélissanne, France, 2015

I came upon Alain Auberville's work on embryology-based motility about 15 years ago, as the young general manager of an osteopathy school in Montreal, the Centre Ostéopathique du Québec. His conscientious clinical work, which integrated the principles of osteopathy, was of sufficient interest to be part of our school's curriculum. Annual classes were offered, allowing us to learn about this work and its evolution.

My personal learning of these techniques required sustained efforts and was not always easy. I wish to warn the reader: in no uncertain terms that the refinement needed to unleash the power of these motility techniques to its full extent is infinite and requires dedication, thoroughness and time. Integrating these techniques into clinical practice must be systematic, keeping benchmarks and references in mind as a way to progressively ascertain their interest and their effectiveness. My experience of learning is very different from that of Alain, which was progressive and experimental. He introduced techniques one at a time both in his mind and in his clinical practice, slowly forming the general concept we present today.

Innovating and introducing new knowledge in a field like osteopathy, while remaining true to tradition and underlying principles, is not always an easy thing to do. In my opinion, the concept of embryology-based motility, more than being a collection of new techniques to add to one's therapeutic tools, enlarges the very vision of osteopathy by introducing a new way of understanding the relations between structure and function. This concept also gives us ways to set out the deep ties between human physical organization and physical, mental, and emotional health. It ensures that clinical interventions will respect patients' integrity by creating an almost symbiotic relationship between the practitioner's hands and the patient's tissues.

Alain's work is so promising and forward-looking for osteopathy itself that, for me, it is of the utmost importance that it can be offered to as many clinician osteopaths, instructors, and decision-makers as possible. Publishing this book is certainly a good step toward transmitting this knowledge to a greater number. I take a great pride in my contribution to a design and editing of this work, and I want to thank Alain for the trust he showed me in this endeavor.

Finally, I wish to thank François Goulet, who agreed to model for the pictures, and Renée Othot, the illustrator, who generously agreed to be a part of this project. The illustrations enrich the content of this clinically oriented book, and although faced with a number of obstacles during their production, Renée persevered.

It is my hope that this book be useful to the reflection, progress, and therapeutic advancement of all its readers.

Andrée Aubin, Québec, Canada, 2015

Introduction

The work presented in this book has been developed over years of experimentation and elaboration by the author Alain Auberville. Originating from clinical practice, the techniques have proven their therapeutic value over time; in fact, hundreds of patients, for whom previous treatments had not proved effective or lasting, have successfully been treated using techniques based on embryological energy.

Although motility techniques are completely different to classical osteopathic tests and techniques, this new concept is deeply rooted in osteopathic principles, and it reinterprets and takes them forward. Energetic- and embryology-based motility tests and techniques are additional tools for the osteopath that, once mastered, will become an essential part of clinical intervention. Furthermore, this concept offers, without a doubt, a new perspective on and understanding of osteopathy.

The motility model, which has been taught for many years, has surprised and inspired both students and osteopaths. The idea for a written synthesis comes from the latter, whom for many years requested it in order to extend and broaden their knowledge. It is now time to oblige.

The book provides an outline of embryology and is not intended to cover the basics of the discipline or replace embryology specialists. Instead, we encourage readers to explore embryology reference books to complement the information outlined here. Because these books do not provide enough information on movement and some aspects might not be covered, we have, where appropriate, included a precise reference in the text. For the most part, we chose to highlight the links between embryological development and the establishment of the final structure by integrating them into the illustrations.

Elements of anatomy and physiology, as well as classical osteopathic concepts, where deemed to be covered by osteopathic professional development, are briefly mentioned or explained, with more advanced notions being covered in depth. We chose to limit our presentation to the osteopathic concepts that are closely linked to the motility model, omitting the other well-known classical osteopathic considerations since they are not superseded by the former.

Also, not all of the propositions and concepts contained in this book are documented by scientific reference; the techniques mostly originate from clinical practice and are supported by it. We leave it to the reader to experiment and take these theoretical and practical considerations further, in the hope that future research might question and improve this model in the years to come. We have included some additional complementary references with the aim of inspiring reflection on osteopathy, its role in healthcare, and possible links to the results of scientific research.

We hope that this work will be the starting point for the development of this new concept and will lead to the discovery of new applications and the strengthening of its theoretical basis. Osteopathy is a practice with incredible potential and opportunity, and we truly hope our contribution might open up new perspectives.

Alain Auberville
Andrée Aubin

Chapter 1

Theoretical Considerations

Summary

The purpose of this work is to define motility by linking it to the embryological movements that shaped all the tissues of the body and to the notion of the energy and vitality of these tissues. This concept of motility, which is faithful to the tenets of osteopathy, will guide our foray into the clinical possibilities.

This chapter outlines embryology-based motility, starting with a general description of the osteopathic field of clinical practice and a presentation of the discipline's traditional principles. The relations between osteopathy and traditional Chinese medicine will also be examined. Embryology, as a theoretical basis, brings a complementary vision of the energetic phenomena used to define health and to understand pain or sickness. Finally, suggestions for the development and adaptation of palpation abilities in the context of embryology-based motility treatments will be given.

This hypothesis can and surely will encourage discussions, reflections, and hopefully, research on yet-to-be-explained bases for osteopathy.

Field of practice and basic osteopathic principles

This section revisits the principle of normal movement for each structure as an important baseline for osteopathy since its beginnings. The consequences of restrictions or hindrance of this normal movement are considered along with their local, regional or complex and systemic implications, and their possible effects on the structure itself.

Established in the late nineteenth century, osteopathy is a substantial crucible for new interpretations of anatomy and physiology from the perspective of therapy. As laid out by Andrew Taylor Still and his successors, one of the great osteopathic principles is that *normal movement of the body's structures is essential to their functions and to effective homeostasis.* Movement, for now, is employed to describe both 'mobility' and 'motility'; these will be defined more precisely later in the chapter.

According to this principle, the local physiology of a structure can be disturbed when its normal movement is hindered or is abnormal (what is called a 'dysfunction' in osteopathy). A dysfunction can be symptomatic, but it is most likely to be quiet in its first stages, especially if the dysfunction isn't too sudden or intense or if it can be mitigated by the organism.

When the body reacts to the demands of this primary dysfunction, secondary modifications can occur in adjacent structures or near the primary dysfunction. These modifications can also affect further structures if they are related to the primary dysfunction via the mechanic, neurological or vascular links inherent in anatomical dispositions or physiological concerns.

If those secondary modifications effectively help in reducing the blockage or restriction on local movement and share the burden of its consequences, while maintaining function and structural balance, the bodily environment will successfully adapt to the primary osteopathic dysfunction. This adaptation, in specific contexts, can remain asymptomatic, although the energy expenditure can in fact be higher to maintain the organism's function and balance.

Given specific circumstances, these new restrictions can become permanent, too, creating new dysfunctions. A dysfunction 'chain' can then perpetuate itself; it can be either short or long, affecting a single system or a whole region.

The organism's response to the demands made on it is never generic and, from an osteopathic perspective, will be modulated according to the number of dysfunctions and their characteristics, as well as in relation to the affected structures. The intensity and chronicity of dysfunctions – as well as an individual's morphology, genetics, activities, lifestyle, habits or background that limits adaptation possibilities – are other variables that shape the organism's response to a dysfunction.

Clinical practice attests that the concept of a dysfunctional chain, with a strictly causal relationship, cannot totally explain the complexity of the organism's adaptations and responses to restrictions and hindrances in one or many of its structures. The correct representation of the body's general balance and adaptive modifications would probably require different concepts used in other areas as well (Davids et al. 2003), such as representing all the organism's osteopathic dysfunctions as a 'dysfunctional network,' 'schemas,' or 'complex balanced systems,' instead of relying only on linear chains. Clinical reality leads us to consider adaptations as truly individual phenomena rather than explaining them with the recurring principles that are often viewed as absolute osteopathic truths.

When a complex dysfunctional network becomes permanent and reaches vital structures (for example, the diaphragm or nervous system), the ability of the organism to adapt is often reduced. Generally persistent systemic symptoms appear on top of already present local symptoms, eventually draining the body's resources and intelligence, limiting the effectiveness of homeostasis and weakening the organism; it is the chronicity stage, in which the body cannot heal and stops responding, in part or in whole, to classical therapy. Literature is extensive on the chronic deficiency stages caused by a physiological or psychological dysfunction while not necessarily linked to any objective pathologic change (Williams 2008). They usually consist of chronic pain, hindered functions of organs or viscera (palpitations, constipation or diarrhea, for example), or extensive fatigue or exhaustion

(Henningsen et al. 2007, Nimnuan et al. 2001). These conditions can affect teenagers and children as well, including babies (King et al. 2011). 'Conventional' medicine struggles with these cases, being considerably less efficient and less able to resolve the associated problem (Tyreman 2010).

Symptoms of these conditions, which can develop into exhaustion and diseases, reveal a lack of general adaptation to emotional and environmental stress. Their nature varies but they are generally intense and linked to the body's regulation systems. Perturbations include sleep disorders (insomnia or non-restorative sleep) or mood disorders. Without being the direct cause or trigger, the lack of general adaptation can be linked to diseases (such as autoimmune diseases or insufficient immune responses, metabolic, cardiovascular or neuroendocrine diseases, or alteration of cognitive functions) and can also increase the impact of bad habits or lifestyle on general health.

Vital body structures and the body's ability to adapt are also affected, without going through gradual alteration, if the organism is under short but intense stress. Decompensation can happen if a stress situation lasts longer than the organism's ability to deal with it, although the organism can sometimes react very quickly when it reaches its turning point.

These osteopathic health and adaptation considerations can be linked to the concept of the *allostatic load*, which describes the organism's processes for maintaining physiological balance by the regulation of its internal parameters according to external demands. Allostatic load is different and more complex than homeostasis, which describes the body's ability to maintain its internal balance only (Juster et al. 2010).

Other consequences arise from osteopathic dysfunction: when restriction or hindrance of normal movement lingers, local modifications in the structure of the affected tissue can be observed, thus resulting in more than just a function restriction. This classic relation between structure and function is the foundation of osteopathic practice. An absence of normal or complete movement can therefore cause many types of alteration in the structure. Some of these alterations can be reversed, at least in part, if the normal movement resumes fairly quickly, but others cannot be restored by osteopathy.

The causal link between the degree of degeneracy of the structure and the symptomatology thus has another meaning. There is a clear, clinical advantage in considering the nature and intensity of symptoms and signs in relation to loss of movement rather than in relation to modifications of the structure. Examination of medical imaging of the vertebral column (Jensen et al. 1994), rotator cuffs (Connor et al. 2003, Sher et al. 1995), and tears of the knee's medial meniscus (De Smet et al. 2008) shows that an altered structure is not necessarily associated with functional losses or pain.

> When faced with a primary dysfunction and its consequences, the body's adaptive response can be local, regional or systemic. When this situation is beyond the organism's adaptive abilities, not only can it become more vulnerable to other stressors, but the effectiveness of homeostasis can also decrease over time and diseases can occur, often signaled by structural changes in the tissues.

The organism's energetic functions

The relation between health and available energy is explained in this section by establishing links between Chinese medicine and osteopathy.

To describe the accumulation of all the demands made on the body experienced by an individual throughout his lifetime, osteopaths use the concept of 'terrain.' The characteristics of this terrain determine the quantity and quality of the available resources when responding to stressors or simply dealing with the passage of time; in other words, these resources represent the organism's available energy.

This available energy corresponds to the vital energy capital allowed to an individual at birth, which includes genetic energy and renewable energy (mainly from oxygen, food, and water). There is a saying that illustrates our dependency and shows a certain hierarchy between these energy sources: *Three minutes without air, three days without water, thirty days without food: beyond lies a threat to life.* Other sources of emotional energy can be added (love and touch), as well as, according to traditional Chinese medicine, other fundamental emotions: joy, sadness, melancholy, self-awareness, anger, fear, and anxiety. Environmental elements are also taken into consideration: light and darkness, hot and cold, wind, humidity or drought, and atmospheric pressure. Some of this energy is used for day-to-day living and maintaining the basic metabolism, reducing the amount available; 'incoming' and 'outgoing' energy must then be balanced to maintain one's health.

As this balance is essential to health, the intention of the osteopath is to optimize energy consumption in a dysfunction-free body with his interventions. He must stop or at least slow down dysfunctional processes by removing declines in, or hindrance to, movement because they otherwise result in excessive energy expenditure, leading to a decline in health or structural pathologies. The osteopath's role is therefore to limit excessive energy expenditure and to encourage the unhindered expression of homeostasis, through considered treatment aimed at the conservation and renewal of vital energy.

It would be logical to consider their energetic functions when treating human patients. Simply put, what is the difference between a dead and a living being, if not that the living person possesses energy and the dead person does not? Between these two extremes, there is healthy life or life with illness. Available energy, considered here in the broad sense, is fundamental to the organism's capacities.

Osteopathy's concern for energy is historically shared by traditional Chinese medicine. The original and most fundamental concept of this centuries-old practice is the energy flow as the center of, and essential to, the body structures' smooth operation. Energy must be able to flow in time and space in an organized fashion, following specific programs paced by hours, days, seasons, and years. In Chinese medicine, energy flow is essential in elaborating and maintaining physiology and homeostasis. A disruption in this flow will cause physiological alterations and reduce homeostasis capacity, and will cause symptoms to appear more or less rapidly depending on the hindrances to the intensity of the flow. Barriers to a free energy flow can cause problems because of energy overflow or depletion. This notion of energy void will be applied to the embryology-based motility concept.

Hence, the flow of energy could be the common meeting point between the embryology-based motility concept and traditional Chinese medicine.

> Osteopathy has a fundamental interest in energy: the quantity available, usage, conservation, and renewal. To ensure a free flow of energy, and prevent or treat diseases, the osteopath removes restrictions or hindrances to normal movement in all structures of the body.

Embryological motility model

This section explains the staple concept of this work: embryological movement as the definition of each structure's motility and a predominant characteristic of normal movement. Relations between motility and mobility, as well as motility dysfunction sources and the importance of renewable energy, are discussed.

Beyond the theoretical demonstration of its presence, what could be the source of the assessed energy that is normalized toward osteopathic therapy? Where is it located and how is it shown? How is it possible to apply the osteopathic principle of optimal movement in each structure to energy?

This work offers a unique perspective on these questions. **This principle is based on the study of all of the body's structures during embryogenesis, and can be applied to every human tissue since no structure stays in exactly the same place after its emergence.** Indeed, all of the embryo's structures move along the three-dimensional axis, from an origin to a definitive position. Energy is essential to the embryonic structure's movement and development as it is the central element of the underlying 'program' that guides the finesse and acute chronology of these movements.

Embryogenesis is certainly the only stage of human life in which all of the body's structures move autonomously, fueled by their own vital energy. This movement is the groundwork of motility and possesses all of its attributes. Primary to the development of all structures, it is also linked to what we could call fundamental energy.

Embryological organization being enduring and constant, the various movements of the structures during embryogenesis apply a direction and amplitude to the motility movements, setting them around a precise axis. Since osteopaths study the characteristics of the normal movement of each human tissue, it is, of course, in line with traditional osteopathic principles to evaluate and normalize embryology-based motility movements.

At first, the perception and evaluation of motility can appear elusive or even chimeric; however, conclusive clinical results vouch for its attainability. Many student cohorts studying this concept have demonstrated that these energetic embryology-based movements and their restrictions can be perceived using gentle palpation techniques, as with any other movement in the body's tissues.

Those primary movements and the associated energy emerge as a fundamental concept in the evaluation and treatment of tissues, as they represent the very vital energy of said tissues. **Embryology-based motility could therefore be considered as an essential part of the normal movement of tissues.**

However, embryological energy does not always show its ideal nature: instead, the motility dysfunctions are the objects of interest of this work, which explores their evaluations and treatments. This imperfect expression can have many causes: since clinical practice shows that renewable energies are closely related to embryological energy, the primary origin of motility dysfunctions would be a bad inflow of those energies, or their inefficient distribution. The ideal energy movement, related to the original embryogenesis movement, must be fed and maintained by the extrinsic sources mentioned earlier: oxygen, food and water, as well as emotional and environmental energies. Their essentiality, combined with the unstable and diverse sources from which they are harvested, makes them the usual suspects when it comes to energetic motility dysfunctions.

Motility can also be hampered by external trauma of various origins: kinetic, infectious, toxic, surgical or postural, all of which frequently obstruct normal movement. Of primary concern for motility is that the consequences of these traumas can also affect, over time, the tissue's mobility because they will not be correctly sustained by their motility or vital energy.

Primary mobility restrictions, when of great scale, duration or significance can reduce, slow or hinder motility to the extent of it seemingly disappearing from a tissue. The dysfunction's gateway is therefore mobility. Under this type of trauma, the structure is sometimes 'inhibited' at first, which can result, if this persists, in tensions of the tissues appearing within weeks, followed by motility dysfunction immediately after. In the acute stage following a trauma, interventions are more efficient if centered on the mechanical aspect, but at other stages, evaluation of the energetic functions allows the practitioner to acknowledge and prevent the impacts of the trauma.

Lack of motility in a structure, outside the signs and specific symptoms associated with it, is very often translated into an excessive density, identified under palpation and signaling an abnormal flow of energy. Sometimes, an energy void can be encountered, but this is usually less common (see the sections on Evaluation of motility dysfunctions and Normalization of motility dysfunctions in Chapter 2).

When evaluating from an osteopathic perspective, and to acknowledge all types of possible movement in a structure, energetic motility should be included as a part of normal movement and systematically added to the bony, osteoarticular, tissular, and classical craniosacral 'micromobility' perspectives (the craniosacral mechanism micromobility concept is explained later in this chapter). All of these movement types should be present for a structure to show an entirely normal movement. **To be declared free of dysfunctions, a structure must be both mobile and motile.**

So, in what order, with what intentions, and how must these normal movement components be analyzed and normalized for mobility and motility to nurture each other and ensure the health of the tissues?

The most logical and relevant first intention is to ensure that tissues can be nurtured by enough energy for them to be as close as possible to normality. This logic, which has been frequently clinically tested, has given repeated and convincing results. The presence of this vital energy is indeed an essential condition for normal motility. How often does a practicing osteopath encounter dense, dry and heavy tissues that resist normalization? How much time and effort is consumed in trying to relax and revitalize them without satisfying and lasting results even if mobility might have been improved by classical interventions?

When suffering from energy depletion, a tissue is still, cannot express its motility and becomes devitalized. In a chronic situation, the tissue becomes dense, dry, cold, and therefore cannot move anymore: it cannot be 'happy' anymore. It responds poorly or not at all to classical mobility techniques, including craniosacral mechanism micromobility techniques. However, the same tissue responds incredibly well to the restoration of its vital energy flow; in a matter of minutes, it can find its elasticity and warmth are back, as well as, shortly after, a quick increase in mobility. These modifications can occur surprisingly quickly even when using energetic techniques for the first time.

Many experienced osteopaths will relate this to their own practices and techniques, even if the models are not the same; their know-how and the movements they have developed, along with their expertise, will often result in the same clinical observations. Studying 'objective' movement parameters or mobility alone will always result in a lack of the qualitative parameters that best explain the tissues' health. The embryology-based motility model has the advantage of synthesizing these clinical concerns into a simple, systematic and coherent set of techniques that can be applied in the same way to every tissue, while being based on a reputable scientific theoretical foundation – embryology – to facilitate learning.

Before concluding this section we will answer two questions frequently asked by students. They pertain to the way embryological motility dysfunctions appear in the definitive structure, and to whether or not these dysfunctions have their direct roots in embryogenesis.

An essential thing to understand is that, even if the underlying principle of the energetic motility concept lies in embryogenesis, the motility restrictions themselves are present in the definitive body; the structures of the definitive body, except in the case of congenital malformations, being in their expected positions and forms, with the energy of embryogenesis having clearly succeeded in following its original path. Thus, the motility dysfunctions appear in a most likely perfectly shaped definitive anatomy. The roots of motility perturbations were described earlier and they do not include the original embryological movement.

Some of the relations between embryological development and movement were discussed by Blechschmidt in *The Beginnings of Human Life* (Blechschmidt 2004). The author suggests that biodynamic metabolic fields and the kinetics of embryological movement are the most important factors in the definitive human form's development – more than the chemical and electrical environments, and more than genetics. According to him, a structure's growth energy is related to its movement, while the movement characterizes development. Finally, Blechschmidt acknowledges the early relation between structure and function, starting in the first weeks of life, and he considers the embryo to be already fully human from a functional perspective.

> The premise of this work is that the energetic motility of all tissues is linked to the imprints of their embryological movements and that this motility is still present and perceivable in definitive tissues. This work is also based on the idea that embryological energy must maintain an ideal flow in a normally formed human being and that it is essential to the health of all tissues. When searching for the normal movement of the tissue, an osteopath must study the implementation of its primary movement. An embryological implementation and a growth plan based on a certain quantity of energy are identifiable for each structure. This energy-laden movement, allowing

> migration and growth, is strictly defined by its axis, directions, limits, and degree of liberty. These characteristics are the groundwork for the clinical interventions on motility presented in this work.

The Sutherland model

This section outlines the importance of the nervous system in Sutherland's model; although it has clinical relevance, its theoretical limitations are explained below.

William Garner Sutherland advanced the osteopathic concepts laid out by Andrew Taylor Still by focusing on the presence of the movement of cranial sutures and by designing the craniosacral mechanism concept. The craniosacral axis is now an essential part of osteopathic training, and we intend to enrich the concept with new ways of thinking rather than question it.

Demonstrating the relative mobility of the cranial bones was the starting point for Sutherland's work. Every osteopath knows the story: the initial instinct when Sutherland faced a disarticulated skull, the dismantling of dry skulls with his pocket knife, and his awe before the articular structures, which together form a perfect mechanism. After this came the first experimentations on humans (on Sutherland himself) and then the development and teaching of a therapy concept which is acknowledged as a revolutionary osteopathic advancement and brilliant application.

Sutherland, while working on cranial articular mobility, discovered that this mobility was rhythmic, dynamic, and originated from the nervous system. It is the cranial rhythmic impulse (CRI). Describing the might and beauty of what he was feeling under his hands, using the scientific methods available at the time, he was already able to suggest that this rhythm came from movement of the brain and spinal cord. He named it 'motility' – a part of the five classical craniosacral mechanism components (which are, as a reminder, the inherent motility of the central nervous system and spinal cord, the fluctuation of the cerebrospinal fluid, the articular mobility of the cranial bones, the reciprocal tension membranes (dural mobility), and the involuntary motion of the sacrum between the ilia).

In Sutherland's model, the nervous system motility transfers to the cranial bones, which then adapt by moving along the three-dimensional axis thanks to the mobility of the cranial sutures. A useful reminder for Sutherland's model is that the cranial rhythmic impulse (CRI) is the driving force behind the craniosacral mechanism, both terms often being mixed up or assumed wrongly to be synonyms. The craniosacral mechanism consists of an alternation between expansion movements (called flexion) and retraction movements (called extension) in the skull. The sacrum moves between the ilia at a pace determined by the flexion and extension of the sphenobasilar symphysis, via the dura mater link connecting it to the cranium. Between the cranium and sacrum, the vertebral column's curves are enhanced and reduced to the same rhythm.

Classical osteopathy describes the impact of the craniosacral mechanism on fasciae, long bones, the central tendon, and other diaphragms. Because they rely on the thoracic diaphragm and deep fasciae, viscera and organs are thought to be influenced and modified by the nervous system's motility at the center of Sutherland's model.

Osteopaths, by tradition and most likely by a language extrapolation, gave the name 'motility movement' to all movements caused by the CRI, but it seems this was indeed mistakenly done, mobility being the possibility of being moved in relation to a place or position, while motility is the ability to move by itself. The classical definition of the craniosacral mechanism states that the only motile structure is the nervous system. All the other structures involved – cranial bones, sacrum and coccyx, reciprocal tension membranes – and all of the impacted structures – fasciae, long bones, central tendon and diaphragms – only bear the effects and consequences. However, they are still moved, even if the movement qualifies only as a micromovement.

Even if cranial osteopathy has been clinically proven countless times, we have to admit traditional osteopathy does not provide a way to directly and efficiently act on the source of the craniosacral mechanism. Adapted techniques were, of course, proposed, but they are based on palpatory experimentations (sometimes having a certain clinical effect) instead of clear explanations. They are also not always based on simple osteopathic principles. For example, some techniques based on the flow of 'fluids' were not backed by key work on, say, cerebrospinal fluid flow, which moves a few centimeters in several hours and not at the speed felt by practitioners.

The Sutherland model raises a lot of other unresolved questions. Acknowledging that the one-and-only source of the craniosacral mechanism is the central nervous system, and that it communicates its movement mechanically via the cranial bones, how can the impacts be of the same amplitude and synced together in the whole body, as the theory states? Wouldn't there be a delay in transmission between the movement of the cranium and its remote impacts (for example, on a lower limb)? Shouldn't there be an amplitude loss in the wave between the cranial origin and the peripheral point of arrival (a phenomenon rarely described in clinical work)? If, as some osteopaths think, those movements are not synced for all structures, how could they originate from the same source? Finally, how to explain the absence of consensus between examiners as to the eventual transmission of the cranial 'wave' toward the periphery? See, on this topic, the Rogers study as a prototype (Rogers et al. 1998) or the Sommerfeld study (Sommerfeld et al. 2004).

However, all osteopaths have already felt, in the viscera and organs, movements intrinsic to bone or tissue structure; it is also a common osteopathic saying that practitioners 'listen' to the tissues. They can evaluate a tissue's vitality with these 'listening' tests, but they are not always on the same page when it comes to the results, origin or significance of their palpatory experiences. Assumptions include the vascular system and/or lymphatic system and/or autonomous nervous system rhythm(s), without any of them giving conclusive results (Nelson et al. 2001, Nelson et al. 2006, Upledger 1995, Perrin 2007). Faced with these persistent theoretical and practical controversies, does the classical Sutherland model really apply when considering all of the body's tissues?

Of course, the Sutherland model remains valid, but its logical application would be for the cranial articular mechanism and the craniosacral mechanism and also their impact on dural membranes, rather than on all tissues. Other effects of these mechanisms, which can often be detected by palpation, will be better explained by the embryology-based motility model; almost all the movements of the remote structures mentioned in the Sutherland model (fasciae, long bones) are the same as those described by embryology. They will be discussed in subsequent chapters.

Since it is designed to intervene on every tissue, the energetic motility model can also act directly on the nervous system – the central element of Sutherland's model. Magoun, cited by Liem (2010), mentions that 'we think that embryological growth movements, in the form of small inherent rhythmic movements, do last, to a certain degree, after the growth processed is completed.' Classical osteopathic practices lack this kind of intervention, aimed directly at the source of the craniosacral mechanism and allowing for its recovery, revitalization, and power restoration. Energetic motility techniques can achieve this with unprecedented effectiveness, and it is then possible to directly influence widespread and common aspects like fatigue states, sleep, cognitive functions, mood, and stress response (see Chapter 4).

Providing a new systematic explanatory model, this work aims to specify osteopathic clinical interventions. The embryology-based motility model, rooting actions in a simple pattern, can describe subtle movements felt by the practitioner's hands in a very efficient way. It also helps understanding that each tissue's vitality is its own, and that each tissue can have its own rhythm and movement expression. The embryology-based motility model does not renounce all the others, but rather completes them with the explanation of the motility–mobility relation.

> The embryology-based motility model's opportunities develop and enhance traditional osteopathy by solving the theoretical and practical problems of the Sutherland model, without discarding this revolutionary model that introduced the cranial field to general osteopathy; it also gives back the word 'motility' its meaning.

Other osteopathic works based on the theory of embryology

Other osteopathic works have their foundations in embryology. Firstly, the model introduced by Barral and his collaborators is a hybrid model based both on some embryological considerations and on tissue-related techniques. These techniques are very different from the ones discussed here, which are specifically related to the energetic level.

Helsmoortel and his collaborators (2010; first published in German in 2002) elaborated a model in which the form and development patterns of organs and viscera are guided by embryological movement. These movement patterns then determine the internal elasticity of the organs and viscera: they named this elasticity *intrinsic motility*, and those patterns do not show any specific axis. Again, the techniques discussed in this work differ from those elaborated by Helsmoortel, which come from another embryological interpretation, even if they can be regarded as complementary.

Oddly, all those techniques were developed for the visceral sphere only, probably because it is very difficult to integrate its motility in the CRI/craniosacral mechanism model presented earlier. If viscera and organs are modulated by their embryological development, why wouldn't the other structures be as well? The model discussed here and its logic apply to every structure, because according to osteopathic principles that apply to all structures, if there is indeed embryology-based motility in viscera and organs, it is also present in every other structure!

Types of pain caused by motility losses

Specific pain with an energetic cause is often persistent and continuous, or at least recurring or more significant at a precise time during the day or during one season of the year. These cycles are often related to the energy flows (daily or annual) described by traditional Chinese medicine.

It is most likely that these pains resist analgesics or anti-inflammatory drugs since they are not closely associated with chemical mechanisms. Specific physical activities or changes in posture bring no significant or lasting effects either because the pains are not of a mechanical nature.

Energetic interventions are efficient and provide a suitable response for these chronic dysfunctions or in any case of resistance to classical osteopathic interventions.

Considerations for palpatory learning

The present model proposes a new component to the normal movement characteristics, in order to evaluate and normalize all of its aspects. To fully take advantage of this new movement component, new specific palpation skills are needed.

Energetic tests and techniques may seem, at first, easy to perform. The osteopath's hand is generally gently applied to the patient's skin and the diagnostic and normalization maneuvers are mostly simple; these will not be the difficult parts.

One of the primary difficulties ironically comes from the apparent simplicity of the maneuvers. Most osteopathic palpation techniques, except listening tests, include a first part based on the practitioner's actions – the motor component of the test or technique. Information flows from the therapist's intention toward the patient's tissues, mobilizing them. The second part is the perceptual component of palpation: the therapist receives information from the treated structures. Information flows from the tissues toward the therapist's cerebral reception areas. Achieving successful clinical results requires the right balance and harmonization between the motor and perceptual components of palpation (Aubin 2011).

For embryology-based motility tests and normalizations, important information is of a perceptual nature only and pertains exclusively to a structure's energy flow. The only motor components of palpation are in this case the guiding or hindering of those energetic movements (see the section on Motility definitions, evaluation and normalization in Chapter 2). The motor actions rely on previously acknowledged sensory information, instead of preceding it as in classical mobility techniques.

In classical techniques, confirmation as to whether the evaluated or mobilized structure is the right one comes from the therapist's motor intention; it comes, in motility techniques, only from the best possible tridimensional representation. This essential representation must include as many of the structure's characteristics as possible to ensure a proper action: direction and amplitude of the embryological movement, of course, but also its precise position in the tridimensional space, its volume, shape, thickness, and so on. In a nutshell, the saying is energy follows intention.

The concentration level plays a very important role in obtaining good results, and cannot be helped or replaced by motor automatisms from repeated application, common in classical osteopathic techniques. In the first learning stages, when experiencing mental fatigue or if anatomical knowledge is not sufficient, a precise mental representation might be hard to develop. The therapist's hand cannot, in these cases, carry on the right information, and clinical reasoning or results may suffer greatly. He or she must be aware of the conscious level needed to be able to judge the intervention's effectiveness.

When learning, sensory information from embryology-based motility must be specifically associated with each structure, thus creating a reliable reference framework. These frameworks can then be used to estimate the possible clinical consequences of a motility dysfunction and the results that can be achieved by applying normalization techniques. With experience comes the ability to examine several structures at the same time as well as to associate interpretation with context. The preciseness of the mental representations can reach unsuspected levels for a beginner, and this is central in the performance of efficient energetic techniques; hence, sustained, constant and extended efforts are needed in the learning stages.

Another important element when starting to learn those techniques is to isolate the new palpatory information provided by embryology-based motility from other already known osteopathic perceptions. Without this special care, sensory receptors will concentrate on familiar perceptions, such as, for example, fasciae-related information. If cognitive confusion persists when it comes to deciphering information related to the new model, results will suffer for sure.

When normalizations are successful, tissues are more likely to open up to all types of movement at the same time because the renewed energy flow allows for an immediate mobility improvement, which can be felt by the hand. The therapist must, in these cases, continue the motility work and precisely decipher all impacts related to all types of movement.

> The refinement and improvement of specific palpation techniques is essential for fully effective and successful embryology-based motility work, even if the techniques can be clinically applied as soon as they are mastered. A high concentration level and a precise tridimensional representation of all structures are needed when evaluating and normalizing; it is essential to develop these skills.

References

Aubin A (2011) Palpation teaching methods: Challenges and issues. OsEAN. Teaching Palpation. Potsdam: Germany.

Blechschmidt E (2004) Comment commence la vie humaine: De l'oeuf à l'embryon observations et conclusions. Paris: Sully.

Connor P M, Banks D M, Tyson A B, Courmas J S and D'Alessandro D F (2003) Magnetic resonance imaging of the asymptomatic shoulder of overhead athletes: A 5-year follow-up study. The American Journal of Sports Medicine 31 (5) Sep–Oct 724–727.

Davids K, Galzier P, Araujo D and Bartlett R (2003) Movement systems as dynamical systems: The functional role of variability and its implications for sports medicine. Sports Medicine 33 (4) 245–260.

De Smet A A, Nathan D H, Graf B K, Haaland B A and Fine J P (2008) Clinical and MRI findings associated with false-positive knee MR diagnoses of medial meniscal tears. American Journal of Roentgenology 191 (1) July 93–99.

Helsmoortel J T H and Wührl P (2010) Visceral osteopathy: The peritoneal organs. Seattle: Eastland Press.

Henningsen P, Zipfel S and Herzog W (2007) Management of functional somatic syndromes. Lancet 369 (9565) March 946–955.

Jensen M, Brant-Zawadki M N, Obuchowski N, Modic M T, Malkaian D and Ross J S (1994) Magnetic resonance imaging of the lumbar spine in people without back pain. The New England Journal of Medicine 331 (2) July 69–73.

Juster R-P, McEwen B S and Lupien S J (2010) Allostatic load biomarkers of chronic stress and impact on health and cognition. Neuroscience and Biobehavioral Reviews 35 (1) September 2–16.

King S, Chambers C T, Huguet A, Macnevin R C, Mcgrath P J, Parker L and Macdonald A J (2011) The epidemiology of chronic pain in children and adolescents revisited: A systematic review. Pain 152 (12) December 2729–2738.

Liem T (2010) Ostéopathie crânienne: manuel pratique. Paris: Maloine.

Nelson K E, Sergueff N and Gloneck T (2006) Recording the rate of the cranial rhythmic impulse. The Journal of the American Osteopathic Association 106 (6) June 106 337–341.

Nelson K E, Sergueff N, Lipinski C M, Chapman A R and Glonek T (2001) Cranial rhythmic impulse related to the Traube-Hering-Mayer oscillation: Comparing laser-Doppler flowmetry and palpation. The Journal of the American Osteopathic Association 101 (3) March 163–173.

Nimnuan C, Rabe-Hesketh S, Wessely S and Hotopf M (2001) How many functional somatic syndromes? Journal of Psychosomatic Research 51 (4) 549–557.

Perrin R N (2007) Lymphatic drainage of the neuraxis in chronic fatigue syndrome: A hypothetical model for the cranial rhythmic impulse. The Journal of the American Osteopathic Association 107 (6) June 218–224.

Rogers J S, Witt P L, Gross M T, Hacke J D and Genova P A (1998) Simultaneous palpation of the craniosacral rate at the head and feet: Intrarater and interrater reliability and rate comparisons. Physical Therapy 78 (11) November 1175–1185.

Sher J, Uribe O W, Posada A, Murphy B J and Zlatkin M B (1995) Abnormal findings on magnetic resonance images of asymptomatic shoulders. The Journal of Bone and Joint Surgery 77 (1) January 10–15.

Sommerfeld P, Kaider A and Klein P (2004) Inter- and intraexaminer reliability in palpation of the "primary respiratory mechanism" within the "cranial concept." Manual Therapy 9 (1) February 22–29.

Tyreman S 2010 Musings on Functional Disorders. Philosophy Psychiatry & Psychology 17 (4) 301–303.

Upledger J E (1995) La thérapie crânio-sacrée, Tome 2: Au-delà de la dure-mère. Satas.

Williams N, Wilkinson C, Scott N and Menkes DB (2008) Functional illness in primary care: Dysfunction versus disease. BMC Family Practice 9 1–8.

Chapter 2

Embryology-Based Motility

Summary

Definitions of flexion motility movement and extension dysfunction, possible dysfunction types, and evaluation and normalization methods are outlined in this chapter.

Flexion and extension dysfunctions: definitions

All the body's tissues can express motility movements or, in other words, possess their own motility, sourced from the embryological movement's genetic footprint. By convention, in this work, the normal motility movement is called **flexion**.

Every motility movement is defined by an axis, direction, amplitude and force. The energetic movement during flexion, in a normal motility state, induces a swelling sensation in tissues; they are filled, to some extent, by this energy flow. The normal movement's characteristics, especially the swelling sensation, help distinguish between two structures sharing an immediate environment. Clinical practice shows that the normal flexion motility movement presents with a slight modulation that can be felt by the hand.

A motility dysfunction, or restriction in the flexion movement, is called extension dysfunction. It represents a deficiency in one or several of the normal flexion movement's characteristics. The extension dysfunction can be found at many levels, ranging from a simple slowing in the overall movement, to a partial restriction, to a complete obstruction of motility. It has to be defined in both quantitative and qualitative terms.

Types of motility dysfunction

The first type of extension motility dysfunction is called energy excess. These dysfunctions cause a buildup of energy in the structures, and they can be detected under palpation because of density. Normalization will aim to regularize energetic flow by dispersing the energy excess and re-establishing the normal flow. They are the most commonly found motility (or energetic) dysfunctions.

The second type is the energy-deficiency dysfunction. This type of dysfunction usually affects an organ or viscera, but can also be found in various connective tissues. This type of dysfunction can have various causes: for example, in an organ or viscera, it can result from a genuine assimilation deficiency, which has to be clinically distinguished from an intake deficiency, or it can also have an emotional origin.

Energy excess and deficiency dysfunctions are often related, as energy flow disruptions can cause both a buildup upstream and a shortage downstream. These disruptions can be linked to the cycles of traditional Chinese medicine: the seasonal or annual cycles (Fig. 2.1) or the circadian cycle (Fig. 2.2).

It is essential to carry out a complete evaluation of the sources of the energetic disturbances in order to avoid engaging in an untimely normalization. As the proverb says, *we must open the window before pulling the tiger's tail ...*

Evaluation of motility dysfunctions

Evaluating motility movements requires the osteopath to develop, as when learning to recognize

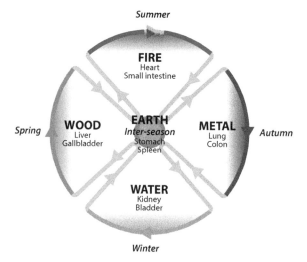

Figure 2.1. Seasonal and annual energetic cycle.

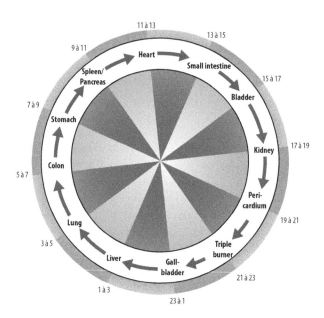

Figure 2.2. Circadian energetic cycle.

movements in cranial bones, articulations or viscera, an adapted palpation technique here referred to as 'palpatory perception.' Two types of complementary tests are used to detect the presence or absence of motility.

First is the **active palpatory perception test**. When using this test, the practitioner has an active intention to verify the presence of the energy flow in a tissue. He initiates the motility movement and assists it in expressing the normal movement characteristics.

At this stage, if motility is completely absent, it is possible to start normalizing, if clinically advised.

If motility is slowed or hindered, it is possible to evaluate the motility movement with the **passive palpatory perception test**, in which the practitioner plays a passive role, receiving, via his hands, the information needed to evaluate the direction, amplitude, force, and swelling sensation of the tissue along the path of its motility movement.

Evaluating an energy excess motility dysfunction

When evaluating a structure in an energy excess state, the active palpatory perception test can reveal anything from a simple slowing, to a partial restriction, to a complete hindering of the normal motility movement. The osteopath feels his hand being repelled by the tissue. The structure seems expanded, overfilled by accumulated energy; the result is an abnormal density, often also found at tissular level (Fig. 2.3).

The results of the active palpatory perception test are completed by the passive palpatory perception test to precisely identify the characteristics of the dysfunction.

Evaluating an energy-deficiency motility dysfunction

A structure in an energy-deficiency state is characterized by a significant loss of vitality in the tissues. The active palpatory perception test reveals a hindered or more often an absent motility, but, unlike with the energy excess dysfunction, the osteopath does not

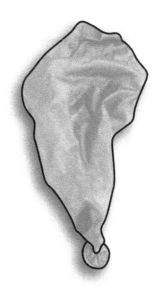

Figure 2.4. Energy-deficiency structure.

feel repelled by the tissue; instead, at tissular level, the response seems rather far away or elusive. The structure is in a state of retraction (Fig. 2.4).

The results of the active palpatory perception test are completed by the passive palpatory perception test to precisely identify the characteristics of the dysfunction.

Normalization of motility dysfunctions

There are two types of normalization for motility dysfunctions.

The first type is called accumulation and is carried out in the opposite direction to the energy flow. This technique involves accumulating enough energy, in the extension direction, to allow the normal flexion movement to resume. In a comparison with road traffic, it would be a blockade that, once lifted, allows the slowed traffic to resume its faster and regular pace. Accumulation is specifically used for the outward motility movements (toward the palpating hand), thus resulting in an effective response.

The second type is called induction – not to be confused with the traditional osteopathic definition which involves PRM – and is conducted

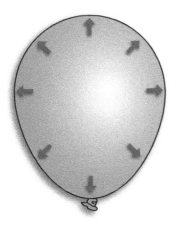

Figure 2.3. Energy-excess structure.

following the natural direction of the energy flow. This technique slowly encourages the tissue to express its motility by actively provoking a flexion movement in the structure; it must, at all times, stay within the real boundaries of this expression. In the traffic analogy, it is like an incentive to drive.

Choosing a technique depends on the subject, the structure, and the characteristics of the dysfunction. In the following sections, the selection of a recommended technique is based on outcomes observed in clinical practice.

Normalization of an energy excess motility dysfunction

Although accumulation techniques can be effective for an energy excess motility dysfunction, induction techniques are used more frequently. Using a combination of the two types of techniques is also possible depending on the context and response.

When structures are in an energy excess state and tissues present a considerable density, special care is required not to normalize the extension dysfunction too hastily or strongly. The use of too much force will add even more energy where an overflow is already present, reducing the possibility of a normalization. These situations require great patience: the 'overflowed' system only needs the smallest possible external guide pointing in the direction of relief, without being forced.

Energy-excess dysfunctions are often easier to normalize than energy-deficiency dysfunctions because dispelling energy is easier than accumulating it in a specific area.

Normalization of an energy-deficiency motility dysfunction

Two options are available when normalizing an energy-deficiency motility dysfunction. First is lifting the upstream blockage (source of the dysfunction; see energy cycles in Chinese medicine). If the blockage is hard to find, great patience is again needed when proceeding with the second option: direct techniques.

Chapter 3

Thoracic and Caudal Plications

Summary

This chapter outlines the main developmental stages of the embryo, with the aim of understanding its general organization, especially the establishment of the thoracic and caudal folds or plications, which are the foundations for motility work. Plications are also linked to the establishment of the diaphragm and perineum and are involved, with lateral plications, in the development of the chambers for the thoracic and abdominopelvic organs and viscera. These theoretical considerations are followed by an outline of the dysfunctions that can affect plications, their origins and significance, and also normalization tests and techniques.

Finally, the osteopathic consequences of dysfunctions of the thoracic and caudal plications on the general state of health and also specifically as they affect the dura mater, the vertebral column, the diaphragm, and the general organization of the thorax and abdomen are explained. This chapter concludes with a note on osteopathic *whiplash*.

The first milestone of an embryo's life, according to this work, is the development of its central axis, which allows for the organization and development of all cells inside the tridimensional space. This 'midline' concept is valued by osteopaths because of its relation with the 'core link' (dura mater structures) and with the central tendon (deep fascial structures). More than a biomechanical function, the midline's freedom and symmetry are associated with the body's general proprioception since an unrestricted and unhindered central line helps to decipher postural information. On a psychological level, self-perception often relies on an unhindered midline.

Blockages of the plications can be the result of an impaired state of health or of an emotional overload. The heart specifically links the thoracic plication to the emotion of joy, whereas the caudal plication is linked to the capacity for embodiment, resonant of its role in the implantation of the embryo in the uterine lining.

Motility work on the embryological movements of the thoracic and caudal plications allows for in-depth interventions along the midline itself. By providing the energy corresponding to its initial establishment, the normalization of this motility then permits more localized interventions on the affected tissues, such as the dura mater and deep fascial structures, with greater efficacy.

This holistic understanding of the body's organization brings new perspectives to some complex clinical situations, such as when localized dysfunctions keep recurring due to their subordination to a superior function (breathing or horizontality of the line of sight, for example) or to homeostasis.

Osteopaths have, for a long time, found 'tough' cases of multiple, erratic and/or chronic pain to be more or less similar: dense thorax with significant blockages and often severe restrictions of diaphragmatic functions, general restriction of the membranous craniosacral axis, and a significant slowing in the cranial movement's rhythm and amplitude. These symptoms often come with a general rigidity of the vertebral column, even if no specific dysfunctions are clearly confirmed. Localized normalization, even if performed carefully, cannot overcome the established complex dysfunctional schemas; normalization of the plications will thus often be the starting point for an original solution.

Certain aspects of embryology help in ascertaining the general organization of the body. Indeed, it is the embryo's plications (thoracic, caudal, and lateral) that allow the development of the thoracic, abdominal and pelvic containers. Links between containers and their contents are already well known to osteopathy, but the chronology of embryological development helps us to understand some of the differences found when the container is formed *before* its contents, as with the thoracic, abdominal or pelvic cavities, or when the container is formed *after* its contents, as with the cranium.

The plications described in this chapter are of primary importance in embryological movement-based energetic work. They are at the center of motility interventions and their proper functioning is an essential prerequisite for localized interventions. First and foremost, plications must be checked and they need to be free enough before moving on with the treatment. 'Enough' can seem rather vague at first, but will become clearer with greater practical experience.

Work on the plications alone will often deliver results for many clinical conditions, but it will most likely be completed by both nervous system work and localized work focused on the reason for the consultation. The motility normalization of the plications is without a doubt a powerful osteopathic tool when treating complex and recurring conditions; it brings a new way of interpreting persistent and/or recurring dysfunctional schemas like those of the craniosacral axis, especially in its membranous dimension, or those of the deep fascial structures.

At first, this practice might seem somewhat easy, but learning to work on an energetic level and taking advantage of all that normalization of the plications can offer might well take months or years of intensive practice. Discipline is essential when learning to work at this new energetic level; and one must not let the hand follow the old familiar paths, as in the instinctive response to fascial or musculoskeletal dysfunctions.

Embryological generalities

These significant events in the embryo's development must be described in order to chronologically establish the sequence of the thoracic and caudal folds (referred to here as plications). These are the first embryological movements to be evaluated and eventually normalized according to the principles of energetic motility.

The establishment of these two folds is preceded by a very complex series of events in which two cells become a full-fledged organism.

First week: implantation

The first week of life is mostly dedicated to the implementation and multiplication of embryonic cells – one of the first significant events in the embryo's development is its settling in the uterine lining. Settling always begins with the sacral part of the embryo, through the connecting stalk. In traditional Chinese medicine, the sacrum represents genetic energy; it is possible to think, after examining many newborns and empirically interpreting clinical records, that the sacrum is related to the newborn's will to settle and then be brought to life. The heart, which is related to the emotion of joy in Chinese medicine, is resonant of the aforementioned situation as it is the first functional organ.

The second and third weeks are dedicated to the conversion of the bilaminar embryonic disc into the trilaminar disc. This conversion then supports many other important events, such as thoracic, caudal and lateral folds, called plications in the present work, which are set to happen in the fourth week.

Second week: bilaminar disc

In the second week of life, the embryo is a bilaminar disc formed by two distinct cell layers, the primary ectoderm or epiblast, and the primary endoderm or hypoblast. It is surrounded by the yolk sac on the primary endoderm side and by the amniotic sac on the primary ectoderm side (Fig. 3.1).

Third week: conversion into trilaminar disc and neural plate induction

Many important phenomena take place in the third week of gestation:

- Formation of the primitive streak and gastrulation;
- Conversion of the bilaminar disc into the trilaminar disc;

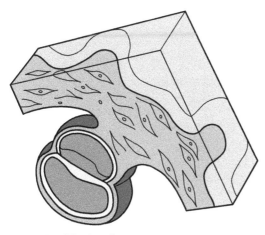

Figure 3.1. Bilaminar disc.

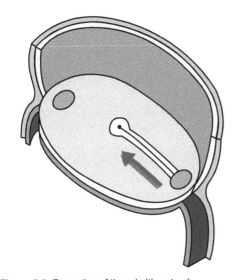

Figure 3.2. Formation of the primitive streak.

- Formation of the notochord;
- Division of the mesoderm into three distinct blocks;
- Neural plate induction induced by the presence of the notochord.

A major event in the embryo's development occurs at the beginning of the third week: the formation of the primitive streak. Its development begins at the caudal end and continues cranially (Fig. 3.2). This primitive streak allows cells to move along a longitudinal axis by providing a bilateral symmetrical plane. The axis then allows for the determination of top–bottom, left–right and front–rear directions in the embryo. Starting from the third week of life, the cell's tridimensional migration organization, originating from a central axis, seems to be an essential prerequisite to the embryo's proper formation.

The primitive streak's formation is followed by the gastrulation process, which consists of the penetration and invagination of the mesoderm by the differentiated ectoderm cells, in the space between the epiblast and hypoblast. The primitive streak corresponds to the invagination of the ectoblast part of the bilaminar disc (Fig. 3.3). This phenomenon occurs in the whole space between the two primitive layers, except along the oropharyngeal and cloacal membranes, thus ensuring their opening when the digestive tract is completely formed. The oropharyngeal membrane opens up in the fourth week, forming the mouth, while the cloacal membrane's opening happens in the seventh week, forming the anus and the openings of the urogenital system.

On the 20th day, the notochord is formed in the caudal–cranial axis from the mesoderm cells that remained along the embryo's midline instead of migrating. After inducing the neural plate, the notochord disappears almost completely, with the only remains found in the nucleus pulposus of the intervertebral disc (Fig. 3.4).

In the third week of life, following gastrulation, the disc becomes trilaminar. The three layers are: the ectoderm, which forms the skin and the central nervous system; the mesoderm, which forms,

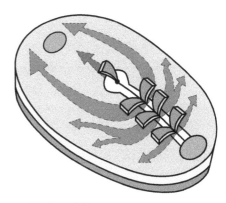

Figure 3.3. Gastrulation.

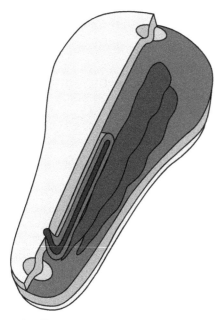

Figure 3.4. Formation of the notochord.

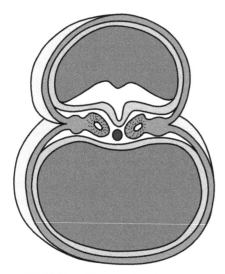

Figure 3.5. Division of the mesoderm into three distinct blocks.

among other things, the musculoskeletal system, most of the urogenital system, the cardiac muscle and the diaphragm; and the endoderm, which forms the digestive tract and the lungs. When gastrulation is completed, the primitive streak regresses and disappears completely.

Once formed as a distinct layer, the mesoderm divides itself into three blocks (Fig. 3.5):

- The paraxial mesoderm which forms the somites, which then divide into dermatomes, myotomes and sclerotomes (see Chapter 9) (Fig. 3.6);
- The intermediate mesoderm, which forms the urinary system and part of the genitalia;
- The lateral mesoderm, which is composed of two plates:
  - The somatopleure, or dorsal lateral plate, close to the ectoderm, which forms somatic or parietal layers, parts of the limb's muscles and most of the dermis and diaphragm;
  - The splanchnopleure, or ventral lateral plate, which lies on the endoderm, forming the visceral layer, the cardiac muscle and the smooth muscles;
  - In between the two plates is the intraembryonic coelom cavity, which forms the future serous cavities: the peritoneal, pleural and pericardial cavities.

The induction of the neural plate and the development of the central nervous system are described in Chapter 4.

The embryonic period lasts for five weeks, starting at the end of the third gestation week and finishing at the end of the eighth. In the fourth week, the organogenesis stage begins, also ending

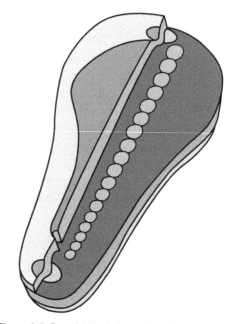

Figure 3.6. Paraxial block: formation of the somitomeres.

in the eighth week. From the eighth week to birth is the fetal stage. During this five-week period, a great plan is in the works and extraordinary events happen by the minute: at the end of the embryonic period, nearly all of the body's structures are already present, although they are not yet fully functional, except for the heart.

Fourth week: folds and formation of the containers

The gigantic cellular development (several million cells a day) happening in the third week precedes and ensures the establishment of the thoracic and caudal flexures in the fourth week, allowing for the formation of the containers and transforming the flat trilaminar disc into a much more complex tridimensional structure, common to the development of all vertebrates. Before the organs and viscera are established, their containers are formed.

During this period, the structures forming the embryo do not all develop at the same pace. Their different rates of growth force the embryo to inflect, inducing the folds. The embryo then progressively takes on its typical 'shrimp' shape.

Folds, referred to in this work as plications, are of the utmost importance for the energetic motility work presented in this book.

The **thoracic folding** process, starting at day 22 and continuing in the fourth week, initiates the delimitation stage for the embryo's containers, especially the thoracic container.

In the first stages of the thoracic folding process, the septum transversum and the multipotent cardiac progenitor cells are located in the superior part of the embryo, on top of the anterior neuropore. They migrate downward from this position, in an anterior tilting movement (Fig. 3.7).

The thoracic fold allows for the establishment of the heart by placing the endocardial tubes parallel to the longitudinal axis of the embryo (Fig. 3.8A).

During this process, the septum transversum is placed perpendicularly to the embryo's longitudinal axis and will form the lower face of the thoracic container. What will become the diaphragm presents, at this moment, a superior concave curve which will be reversed when the hepatic bud appears and grows under the septum (Fig. 3.8B).

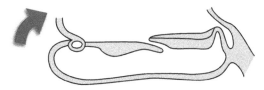

Figure 3.7. The heart's precursors over the anterior neuropore.

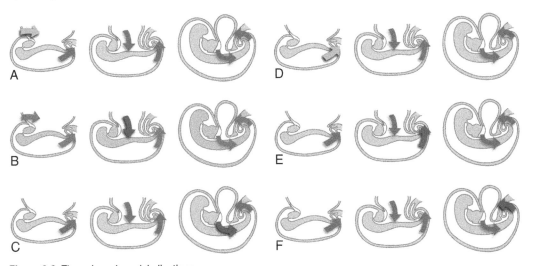

Figure 3.8. Thoracic and caudal plications.
(A) Establishment of the heart. **(B)** Establishment of the septum transversum. **(C)** Formation of the crura of the diaphragm. **(D)** Establishment of the posterior part of the abdomen. **(E)** Establishment of the perineum. **(F)** Formation of the anterior abdominal wall.

At the end of the thoracic folding process, the crura of the diaphragm will be established by a descending movement from the posterior mesogastrium (derived from the oesophagus-associated mesenchyme) toward the lumbar region (Fig. 3.8C).

The **caudal folding** process begins at day 23 and completes its process one day after the thoracic folding. The embryo goes through a differential growth phase in its caudal part, which produces a significant plication of the inferior part when forming the posterior part of the abdomen (Fig. 3.8D). The completed fold sets the inferior limit of the abdomen by forming the perineum (Fig. 3.8E). It then ends by helping in the formation of the lower part of the anterior abdominal wall (Fig. 3.8F).

The thoracic and abdominal containers are completed by the **lateral folding** processes, starting from day 22. Left and right parts of the trilaminar disc join their opposite counterparts and merge completely with the anterior parts of the thorax and abdomen along the midline. In the definitive body, this anterior line becomes the linea alba of the abdomen. Lengthwise, the left–right fusion is complete, except at the umbilicus, where the body stalk and the yolk sac lie (Fig. 3.9).

Curving under the action of the folds, the embryo finds itself surrounded by the amniotic sac. Thoracic, caudal and lateral folds enclose the yolk sac, greatly reducing its opening by restraining it at the midgut. The yolk sac is then integrated inside the body stalk which forms the umbilical cord (Fig. 3.10). It hosts the stem cells to protect them from cell specialization during the embryo's growth stage. Stem cells then migrate inside the gonads when the latter are formed enough to host and protect them.

The lateral closure of the embryo allows for the final construction of the diaphragm from many components. The septum, formed by the thoracic fold, becomes the central tendon of the diaphragm; the ventral face of the diaphragm attaches to the anterior wall at D7 level and its dorsal face clings to the esophagus-associated mesenchyme at D12 level to become the crura; the septum is completed by the pleuroperitoneal membranes coming from the dorsal wall of the body and moving in an anterior direction to unite with it. Finally, the perimeter of the diaphragm is completed by the paraxial mesoderm (Fig. 3.11).

The establishment of the septum during the thoracic folding process explains the cervical origin of the innervation of the central tendon; indeed, the diaphragm receives its motor innervation when 'passing' in front of the 3rd, 4th, and 5th vertebrae. The phrenic nerves then stretch out to follow the diaphragm when it settles between the thorax and abdomen (Fig. 3.12). Adding to the innervation is the paraxial mesoderm, which provides segmented innervation at the diaphragm's perimeter from the last six pairs of intercostal

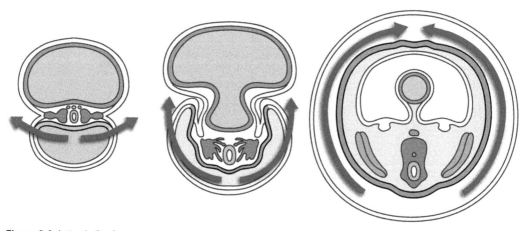

Figure 3.9. Lateral plications.

nerves. Finally, the diaphragm also receives information from the superior respiratory centers located in the brainstem's pons and medulla.

The establishment of the diaphragm obviously divides the thoracic cavity from the abdominal cavity.

The formation of the perineum is linked to the movement of the caudal fold. The perineal body of the perineum is established later on by the cloaca splitting into two parts. The posterior part eventually becomes the rectum and the anterior part forms the urogenital sinus (see Chapter 8).

Following the events of the fourth week of life, all of the embryo's containers, except the cranium, are set. The last weeks of the embryonic stage are dedicated to the development of the thorax, the organs of the abdomen and head, and the viscera, and to the development of the other precursors of the body's structures.

Motility movements and tests for thoracic and caudal plications

The energetic movements of the thoracic and caudal folds are, in the present work, called plications. As clinical evaluation based on the energetic motility concept takes the chronology of embryological development into consideration, motility

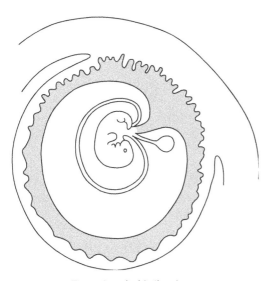

Figure 3.10. The embryo inside the uterus.

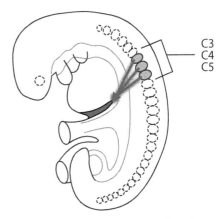

Figure 3.12. Diaphragmatic innervation from the cervical metamere.

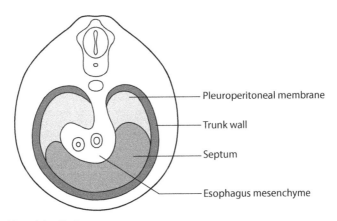

Pleuroperitoneal membrane

Trunk wall

Septum

Esophagus mesenchyme

Figure 3.11. Composition of the diaphragm.

of the thoracic plication and then motility of the caudal plication, are the first two movements to evaluate (see Chapter 10).

To summarize its embryogenesis, the establishment of the thoracic plication is the result of three movements at three different times:

• A descent, which establishes the fibrous pericardium, materialized by the anterior part of the mediastinum (see Chapter 6);
• An anteroposterior movement, which corresponds to the establishment of the horizontal part of the diaphragm (the septum);
• A downward movement, which corresponds to the establishing of the crura of the diaphragm.

To summarize its embryogenesis, the establishing of the caudal plication also consists of three movements at three different times:

• A descent, including the forthcoming sacrum;
• A posteroanterior movement, which corresponds to the perineum's formation;
• A closure of the fold by a circumferential upward movement, which corresponds to the lower anterior abdominal wall.

The thoracic plication comes one day before its caudal counterpart. For an accurate synchronicity, motility movements in both plications must be coordinated and seamless:

• The descent movement in the thoracic fold must be followed, after a slight delay, by the descent movement in the caudal fold;
• The anteroposterior movement of the thoracic fold must be followed, after a slight delay, by the posteroanterior movement of the caudal fold;
• The downward movement in the posterior wall of the thoracic fold must be followed, after a slight delay, by the upward movement of the anterior abdominal wall of the caudal fold.

To feel the motility of both plications, the osteopath puts one hand on the superior part of the sternum and the other under the patient's sacrum. The palm of the hand under the sacrum must be wedged under the apex, on the caudal part of the sacrum. This position is lower than the traditional listening position for the sacrum's primary respiratory mechanism and the contact point is totally different (Fig. 3.13).

The osteopath evaluates whether it is possible for the plications to reveal their motility and thus their direction, amplitude and force. The plications must be *sufficiently* free and motile before going any further with the evaluation and treatment.

Because they come first in the embryological chronology of development, but also because of their clinical importance, plications should always be verified, and verification should take place at the very beginning of the energetic motility-based osteopathic evaluation. Indeed, they provide useful insights on general and emotional states, and they are a good indicator of the predisposition to various important dysfunctions in the body.

Motility dysfunctions of thoracic and caudal plications

The thoracic and/or caudal plication, under a motility loss, is in an extension dysfunction state and is restricted in a part of, or all of its movement. One of the plications might incur a more significant restriction than the other and there may be a lack of synchronism. Plication dysfunctions, varying in intensity, are very common. They are all energy excess dysfunctions.

Typically, when the first part of a plication is hindered, the rest of the movement is also hindered. The intensity of a restriction determines its ability to hinder the complete movement of the plication: a light blockage in the first movements of the plication usually allows for the expression, or partial expression, of the rest, but an intense blockage usually makes the rest of the movement imperceptible for evaluation. Likewise, a major blockage in the movement of the thoracic plication will most likely impair the movement perception of the caudal plication.

Through experience, if the synchronism of the plications is delayed or incomplete, it is sometimes useful to specifically verify and normalize the upper part of the thoracic plication, which can present a significant blockage, largely limiting perception of the rest of the plications' movements (Fig. 3.14).

Modification elements in the perception of movement of the thoracic plication

Without incurring any real dysfunction, the normal movement of the plications might be perceived as modified during evaluation. For example, the

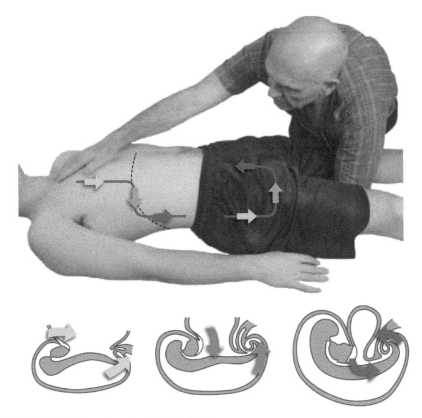

Figure 3.13. Motility of the thoracic and caudal plications.

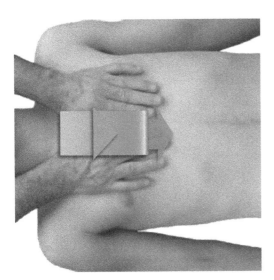

Figure 3.14. Specific normalization of the upper part of the thoracic plication.

related to the septum's descending movement, the pericardium, and the establishment of the heart. Correctly freeing these specific movements can often be useful before normalizing and synchronizing all the other components of the thoracic and caudal plications' movements.

When the entire thoracic plication movement is hard to find, a blockage of the celiac plexus, most likely a significant one, might be present (see Chapter 4). Restriction of this plexus modifies the anteroposterior movement's perception (second part of the thoracic plication) and often causes a denser thorax. When this density resists a correct normalization of the plications, the cardiopulmonary plexus must be verified, especially its inward movement.

Modification elements in the perception of the movement of the caudal plication

Renal motility dysfunctions are common and might unilaterally hinder the perception of the

movement of the thoracic plication is often disturbed by blockages that can get intense, motility of the caudal plication. Evaluation, in these cases, reveals an off-axis caudal plication movement on the side of the dysfunctional kidney. The same phenomenon can be observed in women suffering from an ovarian motility dysfunction (and, rarely, in men with a testicular motility dysfunction), but this source of the dysfunction is less likely (compared to the kidney) and the modification feeling in the plication's movement would usually be weaker.

Bladder and/or uterus and/or rectum motility dysfunctions can also hinder the motility of the caudal plication. Rectum dysfunctions mainly cause an early slowing of the first part of the caudal plication. Uterus and bladder are related to general slowdowns, or slowdowns in the two other parts of the plication.

The caudal plication, even after a proper normalization has been performed, might seem burdened by a chronic intraosseous dysfunction of the sacrum. This dysfunction, especially if difficult to treat, can make it harder for the embryo's implantation in the uterine lining, and could come from emotional difficulties incurred by the mother and/or the child during gestation. Those intraosseous dysfunctions can, of course, persist into adulthood. The osteopath must then take extreme care in respecting this individual's boundaries to prevent raising undesirable and untimely emotional reactions and to make no assumptions of his homeostatic equilibrium, including his emotional state. Patience and deference are therefore the practitioner's best therapeutic tools.

Normalization of thoracic and caudal plications

Normalizing the thoracic and caudal plications is always done in the natural direction (induction).

A complete, or at least adequate, normalization of the thoracic and caudal plications' movements and synchronism often takes time. Patience, concentration and hard work are necessary to gain the benefits of freedom of the plication.

Motility movement and test of lateral plications

To test the motility of the lateral plications, the osteopath places his hands on either side of the thorax or abdomen and evaluates the right and left plication's motility capacity. Direction, amplitude, force and synchronism are verified (Fig. 3.15).

Motility dysfunction of lateral plications

Lateral plications, under a motility loss, are in an extension dysfunction state and are restricted in their ability to join at the abdomen's linea alba, in one or more spots and on one or both sides at the same time. Motility dysfunctions of the lateral plications are less common than their thoracic and caudal counterparts.

Abdominal or thoracic surgeries, as well as traumas, might cause the perception of the lateral plications to be hindered afterward. On the abdominal level, plications might seem slowed by colon dysfunctions, given the proximity of the structures. Lateral plications are less likely to incur dysfunctions than their thoracic and caudal counterparts, and those dysfunctions are usually secondary.

Normalization of the lateral plications

Normalizing the lateral plications is usually carried out in the natural direction (induction).

Links with traditional Chinese medicine

Thoracic and caudal plications allow for work on the Governing and Conception vessels.

The Governing vessel spans from the superior part of the mouth to the back of the perineal body, passing along the vertebral column. It is linked to all of the Yang-type meridians. The Conception

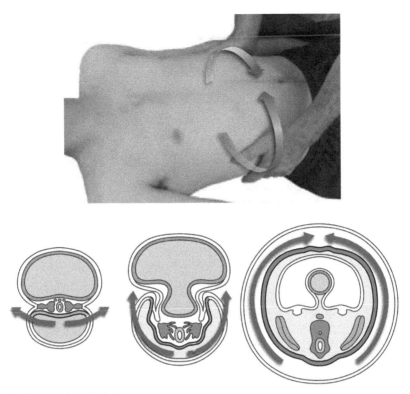

Figure 3.15. Motility of the lateral plications.

vessel spans from the inferior part of the mouth to the front of the perineal body, passing along the anterior midline. It is linked to all of the Yin-type meridians. Governing and Conception vessels encompass the body's vertical axis (Fig. 3.16).

Osteopathic considerations

The normalization effects of the thoracic and caudal plications are numerous and involve the most important structures, from an osteopathic point of view.

Effects on the state of health

Thoracic and caudal plications are the first motility movements to be evaluated according to the intervention protocol (see the section on Clinical intervention protocol for the motility model in Chapter 10). This intention follows the sequence of embryological development, because these plications are primordial both in chronology and in the significance of their role in the embryo's general formation. This significance persists into adulthood, nurturing and maintaining the body's vital forces. Indeed, the plications' movements potentiate the already great effects of the craniosacral system and diaphragmatic freedom. Plications are related to, and take part, whether directly or indirectly, in the general freedom of several essential body structures.

Normalizing these plications frequently results in impressive therapeutic solutions, but although normalization is essential it cannot treat all dysfunctions in the clinical spectrum. Normalizations must be complemented by specific work, especially on the nervous system. They will, nonetheless, quickly become an indispensable clinical tool.

Effect on the dura mater

Work along the longitudinal direction of the dura mater (the falx and spinal dura mater) is initiated

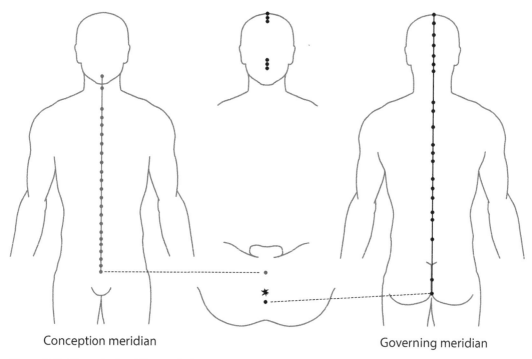

Conception meridian   Governing meridian

Figure 3.16. 'Governing' and 'Conception' vessels.

by work on the plications and completed by work on the cranial folds (see Chapter 4). Dual intervention on plications and the central nervous system gives surprisingly effective responses for recurring and crippling dura mater tensions that are usually resistant to classic osteopathic membranous tissue normalization techniques, both direct and indirect.

The dura mater's normalization in the longitudinal direction is completed by work in a transverse direction on the tentorium cerebelli, which is described in Chapter 4.

Effects on the vertebral column

Normalizing the thoracic and caudal plications allows for general regulation of vertical tension and decompression of the vertical axis, which have a fast and assured effect on the vertebral column's general motility. Repeated clinical experience shows that vertebral adaptive dysfunctions often disappear without any other form of intervention following this type of normalization, although complicated dysfunctions will persist until their

regulation by vertical and costal-specific motility work (see Chapter 9) or more often by underlying work on the medullary level and/or the corresponding neural crest (see Chapter 4).

Effects on the diaphragm

Diaphragmatic dysfunctions, in classical osteopathy, are considered almost exclusively to be secondary to another dysfunction elsewhere in the body or to a postural adaptation. After all, hasn't Still told us that a diaphragm that is able to breathe will do so spontaneously?

A motility loss in the thoracic plication, which establishes the diaphragm, gives a framework for the interpretation and understanding of the installation and persistence of some diaphragmatic dysfunctions that are considered to be primary. These dysfunctions can affect one or all of the parts of the diaphragm (movement of the phrenic center, the crura or the cupolae).

There is also a little known link that explains the diaphragmatic dysfunctions' persistence, without referring to the impacts of the thoracic plication's dysfunctions. Indeed, irritation of the superior respiratory centers (pneumotaxic and apneustic centers) located just behind the sphenobasilar symphysis, might lead to hypertonia of both diaphragmatic cupolae, which is hard to treat with the usual localized mobility techniques, general osteopathic work or even energetic work on the thoracic plication.

Appropriate sphenobasilar symphysis decompression cranial work lifts secondary dysfunctions affecting the pneumotaxic center, while nervous tissue motility work directly regulates primary dysfunctions. The latter often has an almost immediate effect on the amplitude and quality of the diaphragmatic movement since neurologic work allows for a quick response (see Chapter 4).

An unhindered diaphragmatic movement is immensely important for human health. It is therefore a priority to clinically understand the origin of dysfunctions affecting it and to restore its normal movement.

Effects on the thoracic and abdominopelvic chambers

Thoracic chamber

Normalizing the thoracic plication's motility restrictions allows for the specific regulation of the anterior pericardial ligaments. On a secondary level, it also allows for the regulation of all the tensions of the thorax, for the normalization of many diaphragmatic restrictions, and for the relief of many restrictions in the deep fasciae that link the head and thorax. The significance of these restrictions is explained thoroughly in Chapter 6.

Abdominopelvic chamber

Normalizing motility blockages in the caudal plication allows for the regulation of the tensions in the posterior wall of the abdomen by lifting the intrinsic compression caused by these blockages. It also regulates many perineal restrictions when they are secondary to general disorders more than to localized ones. General regulation of the posterior abdomen, associated with the liberation of the crura of the diaphragm and the general diaphragm, has a positive and often drastic effect on the abdomen's general physiology. Presence of the visceral inserts, posterior emergence of the blood vessels from the aorta and the origin of the nervous plexuses can all explain the clinical importance of a proper normalization of the posterior abdomen.

Central tendon analogy

On observing the direction of movement of the plications from a side view, the general shape of the central tendon emerges. According to classical osteopathic theory, this concept links the body's deep structures, from head to coccyx, and also integrates the diaphragms, which represent the horizontal structures. The central tendon concept is often used without any coherent explanation to resolve difficult clinical cases for which classic normalizations do not provide the desired outcomes. When the presence of central tendon dysfunctions is indicated, there are most likely significant blockages, in the thoracic and caudal plications, that are resistant to stretching and postural work, and classic craniosacral work as well. The response to these restrictions will be found much more easily through normalization of the plications' motility than through any other type of intervention. Restoring the plications' motility brings a general decompression of the body's central axis: the diaphragms often get their freedom back by themselves and the thoracic and abdominopelvic chambers are also restored in their proper functions.

Understanding the plications makes it easier to acknowledge the osteopathic saying that claims the cranial rhythmic impulse (CRI) is nurtured by the rhythm of respiration and cardiac contractions, and that working on the thorax region is often a precursor to deep cranial work. Liberating the thoracic plication gives a new theoretical basis to this clinically verified claim.

Notes on osteopathic *whiplash*

In classical cranial theory, osteopathic *whiplash* happens when the cranial rhythmic impulse, at the cranial level, seems inverted in relation to the CRI at sacral level. This phenomenon follows a trauma originating from an unexpected change in the speed at which the body travels; the classic example is a 'full-frontal-impact' car crash.

Although this dysfunctional situation, commonly found in osteopathic clinical practice, is acknowledged, it is difficult to explain how cranial movement could actually be mechanically inverted in relation to sacral movement, as the movements are linked by the dura mater – an inelastic continuity factor. According to the only classical craniosacral mechanism interpretation grid, the only possible conclusion seems to be inversion of the mechanism.

Loss of normal plication motility provides an adequate explanation to this anatomic and physiologic osteopathic *whiplash* problem. In high-speed seated accidents (like car accidents), the caudal plication is very often found to be in an extension dysfunction state, motility-wise. This loss of motility in the caudal plication gives the palpatory impression of a CRI-linked extension movement of the sacrum during the cranial flexion phase. Also, this motility dysfunction of the caudal plication often involves an energetic dysfunction in the left kidney when the accident provoked fear, especially intense fear like the fear of death (see Chapter 8).

Synchronization of the caudal plication with the thoracic plication allows for correction of this perceived inversion of the CRI. The remaining craniosacral system dysfunctions will respect classical osteopathic physiology and normalization techniques are especially effective because they are carried out after proper motility work.

Summary

This chapter focuses on the role that the nervous system plays in clinical osteopathic practice. Osteopathic techniques applied to the nervous system frequently follow work on the plications in general embryology-based motility work, of which they are a very important part. An overview of the embryological development of this system will enable us to understand its entire organization. The structures in need of evaluation and normalization are considered following the direction of the information flow, from the center toward the periphery, a direction usually adhered to in clinical practice. These structures include, in a directional order, the first and third folds of the neural tube, the tentorium cerebelli, the cranial nerve nuclei and the cerebellum, the medulla oblongata and spinal cord, the neural crests and lymph nodes, and finally, the plexuses. This work is completed by work on the cerebral hemispheres. For each of the nervous structures described in this chapter, osteopathic considerations are provided. These describe the important links to nervous structures that must be considered when evaluating the significance of the associated dysfunctions.

In classical osteopathy, the nervous system is only considered in relation to the effects of the osseous and membranous containers on their contents, in both evaluation and normalizations. Although some interesting effects can be observed on the nervous system following classical cranial treatment, for example on sleeping or learning disorders, working directly on the nervous tissue allows for more precise actions and gives better results. Numerous signs and symptoms, previously difficult to alleviate with osteopathy, can then be treated. Work on the nervous system can involve other more systemic concerns related to the general state or information flow, or some more localized concerns related to a specific nervous structure's function. Clinical indications are given in each section of this chapter, but a thorough knowledge of the anatomy and physiology of the central nervous system will lead to satisfying results, enabling the correct recognition, association, and interpretation of the patient's signs and symptoms.

The importance of the nervous system in the craniosacral mechanism and the persistence of the embryological movement in the 'finished' body tissue were anticipated by Sutherland and Magoun, as reported by Liem (2010): 'We think that embryonic growth movements persist, to some extent, as small inherent rhythmic movements even once the growth process is completed.' Embryological movements, especially in the neural tube folds and cerebral hemispheres, do indeed explain the perception of the classically described flexion movement that animates membranous and osseous containers. Hence, the primacy of the nervous tissue's movement, originally identified by Sutherland, is acknowledged in this work, with the emphasis on cranial contents rather than the container.

Neural tube folds are essential elements of nervous system motility work. Their normalization completes the liberation of the dura mater's longitudinal aspect that began with the normalization of the thoracic and caudal plications, as outlined in Chapter 3. Work on the nervous system is also frequently related to the visceral sphere where the liberation of the superior nervous command or the commands of the nerve plexuses is necessary.

Opportunities to work directly on the nervous tissue, either locally or when looking for global effects, are yet to be exploited, but some results suggest a blurred line between structure and function, as in the case of complex regional pain syndrome (formerly known as algoneurodystrophy) that is presented at the end of this chapter.

Embryological generalities

An important phenomenon occurs in the third week of life: the induction of the neural plate from the notochord, which forms the central nervous system. Originating from ectoderm cells, the neural plate is larger in its cephalic section, which will form the brain, than in its caudal section, which will form the spinal cord. This nervous tissue induction happens before the development of the osseous cranium. At the cranial level, the order of formation of the container and the contents is then inverted in contrast to the thorax or abdomen, where the container is formed before the contents.

After the overlying ectoderm thickens as the neural plate, the latter sinks into the embryo during the fourth week, progressively shaping up as a hollow tube by a ventral curvature and closure movement along its median axis. This is neurulation (Fig. 4.1).

During the neural tube's development, some of the cells break away to form independent structures known as neural crests. They are at the origin of several structures, are very different from each other, and are often found far away from the spinal cord (Fig. 4.2).

Spinal neural crests are at the origin of:
- The dorsal root ganglia;
- The sympathetic chain ganglia;
- The prevertebral (pre-aortic) ganglia;
- The adrenal medulla.
  Cranial neural crests are at the origin of:
- The dermis and hypodermis of the face and neck;
- The pharyngeal arch cartilages;
- The aorticopulmonary septum;
- The conjunctive tissues surrounding the eye and the pupillary and ciliary muscles;
- The dental odontoblast;
- The cranial nerve ganglia.
  Spinal and cranial neural crests are at the origin of:
- The enteric ganglia;

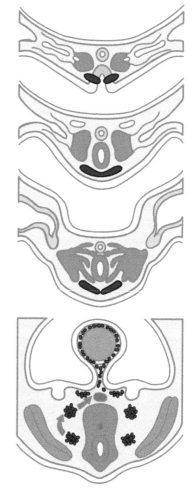

Figure 4.2. Neural crest and ganglia.

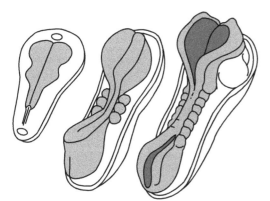

Figure 4.1. Neural plate and neurulation.

- The Schwann cells;
- The glial cells of the peripheral ganglia;
- The arachnoid mater and the pia mater;
- The melanocytes.

In summary, neural crests are the precursors of many nervous structures: the spinal ganglia of the peripheral nervous system, the autonomous nervous system ganglia, the Schwann cells of the peripheral nerves, and other structures further from the nervous system, like the adrenal medulla, the dermis and conjunctive tissue, the internal meningeal envelopes (arachnoid mater and pia mater), and the melanocytes.

In the fourth week of life, the cephalic part of the neural plate, developed into the neural tube, forms three primitive cerebral vesicles. At day 19, the prosencephalon (forebrain), the mesencephalon (midbrain) and the rhombencephalon (hindbrain) are differentiated. During the development of the central nervous system, two of these primitive vesicles are divided: the prosencephalon becomes the diencephalon and the telencephalon, and the rhombencephalon becomes the metencephalon and the myelencephalon, ultimately forming five vesicles.

Between the fourth and eighth week, differentiation in the central nervous system is characterized by three successive flexures of the neural tube in three different places. The first and third flexures, here called first and third folds, are an essential part of motility-based clinical work. Unlike the others, the second flexure has no known clinical interest related to the autonomous nervous system and is therefore not referred to in this work (Fig. 4.3).

The order of events is:
- The first flexure, or first fold, is the mesencephalic curve occurring in the midbrain, which starts in the fourth week and finishes in the fifth.
- The second flexure, or second fold, is the cervical curve occurring in the lower part of the neural tube, which starts in the fifth week and finishes in the eighth.
- The third flexure, or third fold, is the pontine curve occurring in the upper part of the neural tube, which starts in the fifth week and finishes in the eighth.

Building on this general model, the brain evolves quickly. Understanding its embryological development and its progressive specialization is essential in order to apply the motility techniques presented here to the nervous system's structures.

To give an overview of the brain's development, each of its parts is described briefly, starting with the posterior part (cerebellum, pons, medulla oblongata and fourth ventricle), then moving on to the middle part (relay centers) and finally to the anterior part (hypophysis, hypothalamus, thalamus, basal ganglia, epiphysis, cerebral hemispheres). Most of these structures are described and illustrated in this chapter.

Rhombencephalon (hindbrain)

The rhombencephalon divides into the metencephalon (cranial part) and the myelencephalon (caudal part). It is the origin of the cerebellum, the pons and the medulla oblongata, and it houses the fourth ventricle.

The **cerebellum** starts to form from the sixth week, but its development is much faster from the 12th week. The two cerebellar hemispheres grow from the cerebellar plates and merge along the midline. Their growth and specialization continue even after birth. The fast growth experienced by the cerebellum in a confined space makes its surface wrinkled.

In its definitive version, the cerebellum is made up of three cell zones which relate to the diversification of its functions during its development. The most ancient part is the archicerebellum (flocculonodular lobes) that controls vestibular equilibrium. The paleocerebellum appears next, ensuring the tonus and posture of the striated muscles and equilibrium through the modulation of the descending motor pathways. It is followed by the neocerebellum – the most important part of the definitive cerebellum – which controls the automatic coordination of movements and fine motor skills according to information received from the cortex, especially the parietal lobe. Some studies state that this latter part also plays a role in cognition, language learning,

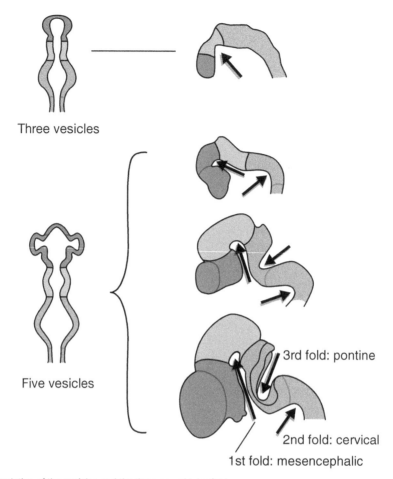

Figure 4.3. Evolution of the vesicles and the three neural tube folds.

attentional and mental imagery processing capacities (Botez et al. 1996, Molinari et al. 1997).

The contents of the **brainstem** are organized into seven columns, divided by the functions of the cranial nerve nuclei. While the divisions between somatic (motor and sensory) functions and vegetative functions are notable in the spinal cord, they are not as clearly differentiated in the brainstem.

The structure of the **medulla oblongata** resembles that of the spinal cord, but the medulla oblongata is home to several cranial nerve nuclei. The medulla oblongata is the relay between the spinal cord and the superior centers. It also houses the nuclei responsible for the cardiopneumoenteric system and some reflex movements. The first

contact point of neurulation is housed by the medulla oblongata.

The walls of the rhombencephalon spread to form the fourth ventricle. The **fourth ventricle** is a diamond-shaped cavity which leans along the posterior wall of the future brainstem. It will host the choroid plexuses, which are responsible for cephalorachidian fluid production.

Mesencephalon (midbrain)

The mesencephalon is essentially a relay center. It contains visual and auditory relay centers: the superior colliculus (vision) and inferior colliculus (hearing), as well as four cranial nerve nuclei, the red nucleus and the substantia nigra. It is related to reticular formation, which continues afterwards into the diencephalon.

Prosencephalon (forebrain)

The forebrain, or prosencephalon, is divided into two secondary vesicles: diencephalon (hypothalamus, thalamus, epiphysis, basal ganglia) and telencephalon (cerebral hemispheres). The forebrain provides the nervous system with its most evolved structures.

From the diencephalon comes the hypothalamic swelling that will become the **hypothalamus**. The hypothalamus controls visceral activity and is related to cardiac rhythm, neurovegetative functions and the secretions of the hypophysis. The **thalamus** also comes from this swelling. Function-wise, the thalamus can be considered to be like a superior sensory center, which acts as a central gateway for all peripheral afferences heading to the cortex.

A ventral outpouching of the diencephalic midline, called infundibulum, will become the neural part of the **hypophysis** (posterior hypophysis). The anterior part of the hypophysis comes from Rathke's pouch, which in turn comes from the pharyngeal membrane initially located near the oropharyngeal membrane.

The **basal ganglia** (putamen, caudate nucleus or corpus striatum) also have their roots in the forebrain. They are analogous to superior motor centers. With the globus pallidus, these nuclei are part of the extrapyramidal system. The extrapyramidal system controls muscular tonus and involuntary movement, while the pyramidal system is related to voluntary movements. The extrapyramidal system's action is completed by the action of the substantia nigra and red nucleus (originating from the mesencephalon and housed in the brainstem in the definitive brain), and by the thalamus. The extrapyramidal system, when affected, causes Parkinson's disease.

The epithalamus, which will become the pineal gland or **epiphysis**, is formed from the roof plate of the diencephalon. The epiphysis, by releasing melatonin, controls the circadian rhythm. It is also related to the reproductive cycle.

Both **cerebral hemispheres** are extensions of the telencephalon. They become visible at day 22. At 16 weeks, they are already large. They develop from front to back, covering the diencephalon. At this time, the hemispheres are linked by a structure that will become the corpus callosum. In the first stages of development, the hemispheres' surfaces are smooth, but their quick growth wrinkles and creases them with complex patterns, giving rise to lobes and gyri. Upon birth, the hemispheres are at 25 per cent of their final volume and weight. They will grow, reaching 50 per cent at six months old and 95 per cent at 10 years old (Cochard 2015, p. 69).

Neural pathways

The sequence of motility work generally follows embryological development but is also concerned with, according to the various reasons for consultation, the transmission of neurological information, either from the center toward the periphery or from the periphery toward the center. Therefore, understanding these communication pathways is important. Below, information conveyed by the autonomous nervous system is considered first, since it pertains to the first embryological movements of the nervous system.

Information coming from the central autonomous nervous center first passes along the first fold (Fig. 4.4A) and then the third fold (Fig. 4.4B). It subsequently passes through the brainstem (Fig. 4.4C). At this level, parasympathetic information from the brainstem nuclei departs toward the target organs. Orthosympathetic information continues to the medulla oblongata, spreading in the spinal cord (Fig. 4.4D). It emerges at the periphery via the ganglia located at spinal and costal level (Figs 4.4E, F). For viscera and organs, it is necessary to consider the nerve plexuses (Fig. 4.4G) of the arterial trunks (Fig. 4.4H) and the enteric ganglia located in organs and viscera walls (Fig. 4.4I) to complete the routing of information from a central origin to its target organ. Orthosympathetic information is completed by parasympathetic information coming from the sacral region for the distal colon and the pelvic cavity organs (not illustrated here).

In the opposite direction, peripheral information coming from viscera and organs as well as from the musculoskeletal system's structures can influence the nervous system, either via segmental effect or by going to the superior centers. The even closer relationship between the nervous and digestive systems is described in Chapter 7.

Several components of the nervous system are described and detailed below. In principle, the same motility work can be applied to all structures of the nervous system, but the structures presented here are the most commonly encountered in clinical practice. The importance of the information's neural pathway is reviewed in Chapter 10.

First neural tube fold

The first and third folds are related to the orthosympathetic component of the autonomous nervous system. This orthosympathetic component is in turn related to energy expenditure and to the control of vascularization of all the body's

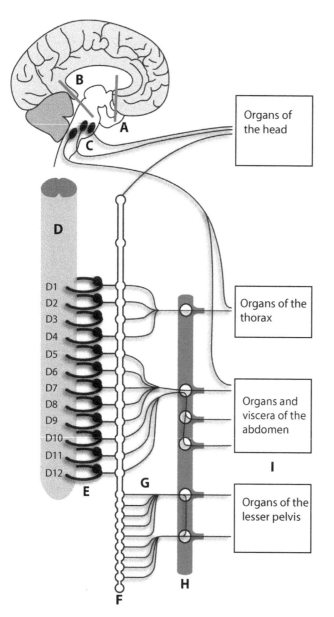

A. First fold
B. Third fold
C. Brain stem
D. Spinal cord
E. Spinal ganglia
F. Sympathetic chain ganglia
G. Plexus organization
H. Aorta and arteries
I. Organs, viscera and enteric ganglia

Figure 4.4. Disposition of the neural pathways of the autonomous nervous system between center and periphery. **(A)** First fold. **(B)** Third fold. **(C)** Brain stem. **(D)** Spinal cord. **(E)** Spinal ganglia. **(F)** Sympathetic chain ganglia. **(G)** Plexus organization. **(H)** Aorta and arteries. **(I)** Organs, viscera, and enteric ganglia.

tissues. It is also linked to diurnal activities and luminosity.

Embryological movement

The first neural tube fold is established by the fourth week in what will eventually become the midbrain. This first fold has great amplitude and allows for the establishment of the orthosympathetic nuclei, which are situated in the medial part of the hypothalamus. Among other functions, the orthosympathetic nuclei are responsible for the regulation of the heart, the first functional organ of the embryo, which is why this fold is established at such an early stage in the embryo's development.

Motility movement and test

During the movement that establishes the first fold, the neural tube folds around a transversal axis in the mesencephalic region of the brain. The neural tube moves from bottom to top with in a movement of great amplitude.

To assess the first fold's motility, the osteopath places his hands on both sides of the cranium, at the level of the sella turcica in the definitive cranium. From this reference point, he creates a virtual axis between his two hands to evaluate the width and height of the global movement of the first neural tube fold.

The only thing to consider while performing this test is the primitive neural tube's embryological movement at its formation, and not the subsequent development of the brain and surrounding structures (Fig. 4.5).

Motility dysfunction

The first fold, under a motility loss, is in an extension dysfunction state and is restricted in its upward movement. These restrictions need to be checked carefully because their amplitude, localization, and qualitative characteristics provide a variety of information for their interpretation according to clinical context.

The first fold may suffer from blockages of its global movement (bilateral extension) varying in amplitude or from one or several unilateral restrictions, located in precise points along the neural tube's width and varying in intensity.

A first fold in a **bilateral extension** dysfunction state implies an impairment of function in the orthosympathetic part of the autonomous nervous system. The bilateral extension dysfunction usually comes from a conscious response to stress, unlike with the third fold where this is usually associated with an unconscious response. The intensity of the loss of normal bilateral movement in the first fold usually matches the intensity of the impairment of function in the autonomous nervous system (see Links with the autonomous nervous system, in the Osteopathic considerations section of the present chapter).

A first fold in a unilateral extension dysfunction state involves a rather precise movement restriction located between the fold's periphery and its central axis. This dysfunction usually comes from an impairment of function in an ipsilaterally located viscus or organ (see Links with the visceral sphere later in this chapter).

While verifying the motility movement of the first fold, it is also possible to specifically evaluate potentially existing tensions in the walls. Without entering into an exhaustive description, it is useful to know that the anterior wall is linked to the various nuclei of the hypothalamus and to the neurohypophysis (see Chapter 5) and that the posterior wall is linked to the respiratory centers and, in a broader way, to the reticular formation.

It is, of course, possible to encounter several different combinations of dysfunctions in the first fold; these will be unveiled by the normalization process since one dysfunction can hide behind another.

Normalization

Staying in the test position, the osteopath builds the first fold's virtual axis between his two hands. He then moves the axis in the cephalic direction, going directly against the encountered restriction(s) until the entire fold regains the best possible motility. He strives for a better movement

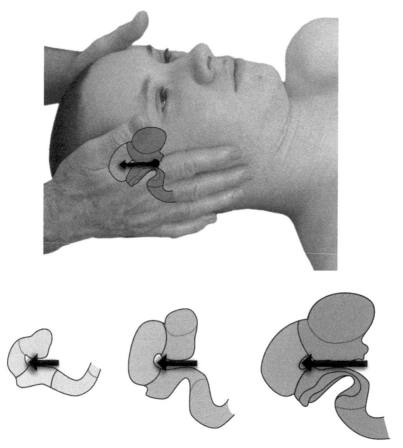

Figure 4.5. Motility of the first neural tube fold.

along the fold's entire width and for the entire potential height of the upward movement. Motility techniques in the natural direction, or induction, are always used to normalize the first fold.

Osteopathic considerations

Bilateral extension: links with the autonomous nervous system

The orthosympathetic nuclei of the medial part of the hypothalamus are located in the central zone of the first fold during its formation. They are functionally related to stress management by their orthosympathetic role. Since stress, in an organism, does not generate constant effects, it has to be regulated for the organism to provide a suitable response, in the pursuit of a homeostatic state. Stress response is extremely variable from one individual to another, but also for the same individual in different circumstances or moments. Clinically speaking, links between stress and the consulting patient's state have to be established with care. The osteopath, depending on his speciality and mandate, prioritizes the information sourced from palpation.

The stress response stages described here are related to the intensity of the clinically encountered bilateral extension blockages found during motility evaluation of the first fold:

• **Stage 1:** when stress is duly managed or dealt with according to existing resources, the functional equilibrium between the orthosympathetic and parasympathetic parts of the autonomous nervous system is observed, and the whole of the first fold is generally free.

- **Stage 2:** when stress is poorly managed or there is a deficit in the individual's capacity to adapt, hypersympatheticotonia appears and the functional equilibrium between the orthosympathetic and parasympathetic parts of the autonomous nervous system starts to be disrupted. It is tougher for the individual to recover and its energetic reserves can gradually dwindle; it is also tougher to fall asleep. Reducing the sources of stress or managing them better is necessary. The entire first fold usually starts to lose amplitude. The ease of normalization for this extension dysfunction depends on variables such as its duration and its relation to a stressful current or ancient situation. It should not be assumed that liberation will be quick or easy, and it is necessary to adapt to the characteristics of the upward movement restriction and to respect the tissues.

- **Stage 3:** when stress is either too intense or extended for an individual's resources, hypersympatheticotonia becomes severe. The individual can have serious difficulty falling asleep and drowsiness often occurs, regardless of actual rest. The movement's amplitude loss in the entire first fold is usually greater. As in the second stage, the ease of normalization varies, but it generally takes longer to reach it.

- **Stage 4:** building on stage 3, if the stress persists or worsens, hypersympatheticotonia can become an orthosympathetic inhibition, leading to a relative hyperparasympatheticotonia caused by the collapse of the orthosympathetic function. Together with the sleep disorders mentioned in stage 3, this situation might lead to phenomena pertaining to hyperparasympatheticotonia, such as a vasovagal attack, a drop in blood pressure, repeated asthma attacks, sudden perforated ulcer, etc. Individuals in stage 4 are generally in a more or less intense state of exhaustion. In these cases, the entire first fold movement is usually in complete extension and the structure is incapable of any upward movement. A complete extension is often very hard or even impossible to normalize

in one session, even if the session is entirely dedicated to this.

These stages are also related to the organism's physiological responses to stress as described in the allostatic charge theory (Juster et al. 2010). This theory describes the behavior of the sympathetic–adrenal–medullatory (SAM) and hypothalamic–pituitary–adrenal (HPA) axis, supervised by the brain (hippocampus, amygdala and prefrontal cortex), when solicited by stress factors. Allostatic charge also describes how the needs, responses, and resilience of the organism under stress are influenced by individual differences such as genetics, life habits, and previous history (environment, traumas, major life events). Further research would provide interesting insights into the links between clinical results from the aforementioned normalizations of the autonomous nervous system and more precise observations of different allostatic charge indicators.

The autonomous nervous system is an extremely complex regulation system that acutely governs responses to the body's management of its energetic resources. It is useless to consider osteopathic intervention possibilities for this system without taking its complexity and the body's own intelligence into account. Hence, those descriptions have to be adapted to therapeutic reality. Clinically, when encountering significant restrictions in the first fold's movement, the autonomous nervous system loses part of its capacity to adapt, which reduces its ability to regulate the body in general. Precise embryological motility work on the cranial folds is a very powerful way to win this capacity to adapt back, when it has been lost due to intense and/or extended stress responses.

Apart from unusual exceptions, evidence of parasympatheticotonia is nearly always an indication of a malfunction, or even a collapse, of the orthosympathetic function of the autonomous nervous system. The autonomous nervous system's physiology suggests that restoring its functional capacity is done through the orthosympathetic function, by normalizing of the first fold.

Working on the orthosympathetic nuclei of the medial part of the hypothalamus, which control the vasoconstriction of all arterial, venous and lymphatic vessels, allows for a possible general effect on circulation when normalizing the first fold. It is often illusory or totally impossible to apply the osteopathic arterial law without bringing the autonomous nervous system's functions into the therapeutic equation, since it controls the entire vascular system.

Note the interesting clinical connections relating to the order in which the container and contents of the head are established. As stated before, the contents, at the cranial level, are established before their container. This primacy of movement of the contents being essential for the entire mechanism's function is also found in the concept of the classical craniosacral mechanism. When the primary problem is related to the motility of the contents of the cranium, classical cranial work might not lead to satisfactory results, unlike embryology-based motility normalization, which provides much more interesting answers. Classical articular and membranous work, when following motility work on the contents, can be of a much greater effectiveness.

For example, the extension dysfunction of the sphenobasilar symphysis is classically associated with the organism's needs regarding regulation, but its localized correction is often of no interest, having a very limited therapeutic effectiveness. Introducing the first fold of the nervous system into the equation helps in the understanding of how motility restrictions in the upward movement can be a likely source of mechanical extension dysfunctions in the sphenobasilar symphysis and how they explain the classically described impacts. It is then easy to achieve a generally spontaneous normalization of the articular extension of the sphenobasilar symphysis with energetic motility work on the first fold.

Especially when used alongside other interventions on the nervous system (see the sections Third fold of the neural tube and Parasympathetic component of the first fold: lateral expansion, in this chapter), working on the first fold gives the opportunity to free many cranial, articular, and membranous mechanical tensions that are seemingly subordinate to the former. The first fold is related to general cranium tensions, especially in the anterior cranial sphere; the third fold is more precisely related to the posterior cranial sphere.

Unilateral extension: links with the visceral sphere

The first fold area seems to clinically be the place where intense and/or repeated nociceptive information from the visceral sphere increases the impact on the nervous system by causing specific neural tissue motility deficiency. Mapping the effects of this visceral information on the first fold was done empirically from extensive clinical experience. The nervous pathways uniting the digestive system and the central nervous system are described in Chapter 8, but existing knowledge on this topic is not sufficient to precisely describe which pathways are involved in the clinical propositions (Fig. 4.6).

An extension dysfunction of the central part of the first fold alone is related to information fed to the central nervous system by the heart, the thymus and thyroid, the pancreas, and the small intestine.

An extension dysfunction of a part of the left side of the first fold is related to, from left to center, information fed to the central nervous system by the kidney, the lung or the left part of the colon, the spleen, the stomach, and the esophagus.

An extension dysfunction of a part of the right side of the first fold is related to, from right to center, information fed to the central nervous system by the kidney, the lung or the right part of the colon, the liver, and the gall bladder.

When information of visceral origin is registered in neural tissue, it can cause pattern reflex activity, explaining some relapses after an adequately applied visceral osteopathic treatment. As a matter of fact, remnants of an organic dysfunction may persist in the first fold's nervous tissue even when the signs and symptoms of the original visceral dysfunction have disappeared or have healed locally. This phenomenon is probably caused by the same mechanism responsible for the 'phantom' pain caused by chronic irritation of the neural tissue.

In the most extreme cases, chronic neurological irritation becomes primary and severely affects the functioning of organs and viscera. Losing their neurological 'nurture' and lacking regulation, they become 'empty' – a recognized concept of Chinese medicine as referred to in Chapter 1. In these

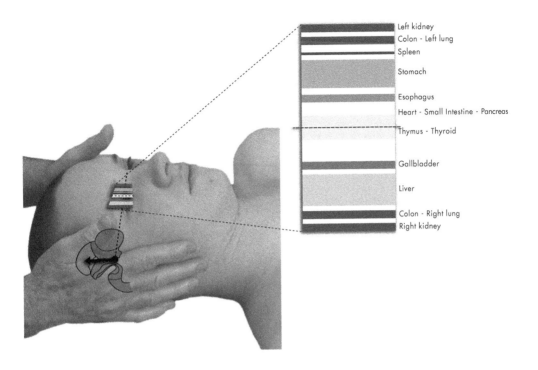

Left kidney
Colon - Left lung
Spleen
Stomach
Esophagus
Heart - Small Intestine - Pancreas
Thymus - Thyroid
Gallbladder
Liver
Colon - Right lung
Right kidney

Figure 4.6. Visceral relations of the first fold.

situations, localized normalizations are particularly ineffective and can even be aggravating. Before aiming for a lasting correction in an organ or viscus suffering from a deficiency dysfunction, it is necessary to start by treating the first fold's nervous tissue that is specifically linked to the concerned organ or viscus. In this situation, energetic motility work provides an additional level of work in order to understand the position, persistence and normalization of visceral dysfunctions; it has to be integrated into the therapeutic approach. An indicator for a dysfunction of an energetic origin is a pain that is generally constant, that does not vary in the same way to the same conditions (like exercise or rest) and that does not react in the expected way to traditional normalization techniques or to medication.

When the unilateral dysfunction of the first fold cannot be corrected sufficiently, it is necessary to check the organ or viscus in order to compare the intensity of the localized and central blockages. The more significant restriction is usually the one to prioritize. If nociceptive information is still active at organic level, relieving the first fold in an effective way will often be very hard. If the central

neurological irritation compromises the visceral correction, an alternation of localized visceral work and neurological work should sometimes be used for a proper regulation of the dysfunctions and to find a long-term solution to the reason for consultation. In these cases, a progressive improvement in visceral and neural tissue dysfunctions implies that the 'alternation' solution is working.

It is possible that visceral dysfunctions uncovered by osteopathic evaluation could mostly have an emotional origin (see emotional links for each organ or viscus according to traditional Chinese medicine in subsequent chapters). Normalizing the first fold is, of course, easier when the emotional problem is past and resolved than when it is related to current perturbations of the organ or viscus.

Links with the superior respiratory centers

Since the superior respiratory centers (pneumotaxic and apneustic) are related to the first fold, normalizing the latter can improve the inspiration superior command function for the diaphragm. More freedom and amplitude of movement is found in the entire diaphragmatic function (phrenic center, and then diaphragmatic cupola) following the normalization of the first fold (see Chapter 3). Functional losses in the diaphragm are scarcely explained by mechanical blockages or localized neurological restrictions (the last six intercostal nerves and/or the cervical metameric level), and they find sustainable solutions in neurological work on the superior centers.

Links with medication

Central nervous system medication intake is not easy to dose and clinical experience shows that energetic work on the nervous system, especially on the first fold, often makes medication more effective, most likely because a better motility makes for a better assimilation. Individuals suffering from Parkinson's disease have seen their medication intake become easier to manage following this type of treatment. Antidepressants also seem to have been, in many cases, more effective following an intervention that returned normal movement capacities to the first fold and to the central nervous system in general.

Caution: contraindication

The normalization of the first fold must be applied with caution during pregnancy because, when liberating superior respiratory centers, the implied relaxation of the diaphragm may cause the uterus to take a more posterior position, which can then sometimes hinder the inferior vena cava and cause vagal discomfort.

Third neural tube fold

Embryological movement

The third fold is the pontine flexure occurring in the lower part of the neural tube's cephalic part.

Motility movement and test

To evaluate the third fold's motility, the osteopath places one hand at the level of the inion on the squamous part of the occipital bone in the definitive cranium. From there, he creates the virtual axis of the third fold and evaluates the folding movement of the neural tube in the caudal part of the primitive brain (in the infratentorial region). To help represent it, this complete motility movement can be seen as following the shape of the squamous part of the occipital bone.

The first information coming from the central inion contact point pertains to the central and posterior parts of the fold. Pursuing the work toward the front end, information pertaining to the lateral parts of the neural tube fold is progressively revealed.

The only thing to consider while performing this test is the embryological movement of the primitive neural tube as it establishes itself, and not the brain's subsequent developments (Fig. 4.7).

Motility dysfunction

The third fold, under a motility loss, is in an extension dysfunction state and the amplitude of its movement is restricted.

The third fold may suffer from blockages of its global movement, varying in intensity, or from a unilateral restriction. As with the first fold, the third fold, in an extension dysfunction state, implies an impairment of function in the orthosympathetic part of the autonomous nervous system, because the third fold's role is to transmit information from the hypothalamus' orthosympathetic nuclei to the cranial nerve nuclei and to the spinal cord. It is essential, following work on the first fold, to pay attention to the third before moving onto the peripheral structures.

The bilateral extension intensity of the movement may also match the intensity of the impairment of function.

The third fold's movement restriction can be related to unconscious stress response or to the emotional aspect. Thus, it is often linked to

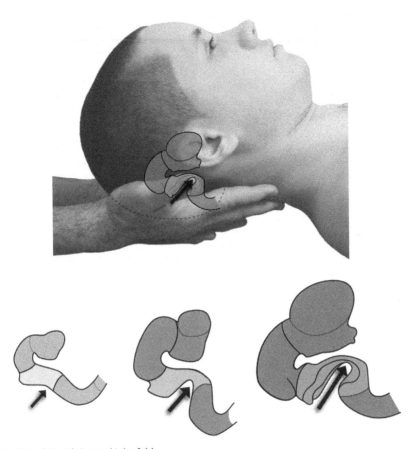

Figure 4.7. Motility of the third neural tube fold.

intense and/or chronic thoracic tension of the pericardial ligaments and/or the fibrous pericardium itself. A sustained extension of the third fold can then be linked to a compression of the cervical region, stuck between simultaneous thoracic and cranial tensions.

Unilateral restrictions in the third fold, unlike their counterparts in the first fold, are difficult to identify specifically; their normalizations are usually carried out in a more general and broad manner than normalizations of the first fold.

Normalization

Remaining in the test position, the osteopath creates the third fold's virtual axis in his palms at the level of the inion. He then moves the axis toward the infratentorial region. This movement can be seen as following the squamous part of the occiput's movement during flexion of the spheno-basilar articulation. The osteopath normalizes against the restriction until the best possible motility is restored. As with the first fold, motility techniques in the natural direction, or induction, are always used to normalize the third fold.

Osteopathic considerations

Links with the autonomous nervous system

Because it transmits information from the center to the periphery, the first fold's movement must be free enough before starting to work on the third; work on both folds must be seen as complementary.

Extension dysfunction of the first fold implies typical sleep disorders (difficulty falling asleep); conversely, when a significant extension of the third fold is present, sleep is often ineffective and people feel as tired when they wake in the morning as they did when going to bed the night before. When significant dysfunctions are found in both the first and third folds, sleep is often impaired in all possible ways and has been for a long time.

Links with the cranial mechanism

Usually, since it is closely linked to the occiput, the third fold is mostly associated with the posterior cranial sphere. For example, the third fold may be related to types of tinnitus, especially those that vary in intensity and that show vascular and nervous characteristics.

Caution: contraindication

Neurological work on the superior centers must be used with care during pregnancy, especially if there are already signs of work or spontaneous abortion risks. Work on the posterior zone (the third fold) seems to come with many drawbacks, probably because of its possible side effects on the cranial nerve nuclei known to be, according to osteopathic tradition, sensitive to the use of the fourth ventricle compression technique (CV4).

Osteopathic considerations for combined first- and third-fold work

As discussed in the section on plications, the normalization of the two folds plays a very important role in the freedom of the longitudinal component of the dura mater. While normalizing the plications initiates the general decompression work on the body's central axis, work on the folds, because it restores freedom to the contents of the cranium (thus freeing the container), completes the normalization of the dura mater's longitudinal aspect. Work in the transverse direction is sometimes necessary for the complete liberation of this system (see the section on Tentorium cerebelli).

The freedom of the dura mater is an essential prerequisite for the normalization of compressions affecting the vertebral column and sometimes the inferior limbs (see Chapter 9). The dura mater's general significance is well-known to classical osteopathy.

Parasympathetic component of the first fold: lateral expansion

The lateral expansion that occurs at the end of the first fold's movement is linked to the parasympathetic component of the autonomous nervous system responsible for restoration (rest) of energetic resources and for cellular repairs. The parasympathetic component is also linked to the nocturnal phase of the circadian rhythm and to darkness.

Embryological movement

In the first fold, the parasympathetic nuclei of the hypothalamus are laterally located by the sympathetic nuclei. In the chronological sequence of embryological development, their establishment occurs just after that of the orthosympathetic nuclei.

The motility of the autonomous nervous system's parasympathetic component consists of a lateral expansion movement that occurs at the very end of the amplitude of the upward movement in the first fold. In the classical concept of cephalorachidian fluid fluctuations, this relationship between transversal fluctuations and the parasympathetic system is present, although not precisely explained.

Motility movement and test

The test is the same as with the first fold, but the osteopath specifically looks for a lateral expansion at the end of the upward movement. The first fold's movement has to remain free for this expansion movement to be felt. A complete ascent of the first fold, relating to the orthosympathetic part of the autonomous nervous system, followed by an ample lateral expansion, relating to the parasympathetic part, constitutes the proper functioning and physiology of the autonomous nervous system (Fig. 4.8).

Bilateral dysfunctions are mostly related to impairments of function in the autonomous nervous system.

Unilateral dysfunctions are often caused by same-side restrictions in the container, the tentorium cerebelli or the temporal bone. Lifting these restrictions is necessary to achieve full transversal motility, because they often prevent the complete normalization of the nervous tissue.

Motility dysfunction

The parasympathetic component of the first fold, under a motility loss, is in an extension dysfunction state and is restricted in its lateral expansion movement, which usually occurs at the end of the first fold's upward movement. This lateral expansion restriction can be bilateral or unilateral.

Normalization

Liberating the parasympathetic component linked to the cranium's transversal aspect is mostly done spontaneously after liberating the first and third folds (or the orthosympathetic part of the autonomous nervous system). Thus, specific clinical indications for this normalization are rather unusual.

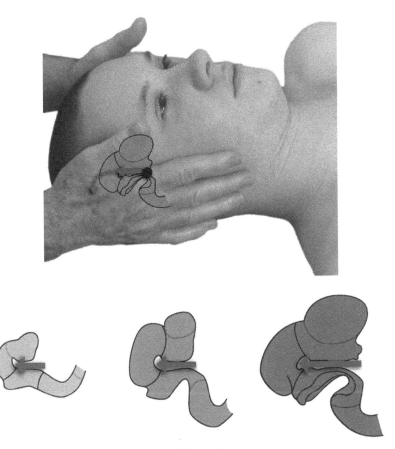

Figure 4.8. Motility of the parasympathetic component of the first fold.

After normalizing the first fold, an indirect technique may be used to achieve the specific normalization of the parasympathetic component. Indirect techniques, or accumulation, are not usually used on the cranium, but they do work in this case. This normalization is performed by applying pressure in the direction of the lateral expansion to accumulate energy, which then facilitates liberation. It is also possible to follow the natural direction (induction) by gently inducing the lateral expansion at the end of the first fold's possible amplitude.

If a bilateral restriction in the lateral expansion persists after liberating the first fold in the most complete way possible, working on the third fold before coming back to the transversal restriction might be an interesting option.

Osteopathic considerations

A unilateral transversal restriction can be linked to a parasympathetic disorder in an organ or viscus located on the same side. If the restriction is easy to lift, the visceral dysfunction is most likely due to a nervous command disorder or to a deficiency caused by inefficient assimilation. When the restriction is harder to lift, the visceral dysfunction might be more significant and checking for a pathology or a primary deficiency may prove useful. If in doubt, refer to a physician.

Tentorium cerebelli

Where possible, energetic membranous work on the tentorium cerebelli is easier and more useful after complete lateral expansion at the end of the upward movement of the first fold is possible (or consequently, after completely liberating the folds of the central nervous system).

Because of the proximity of the free border of the tentorium cerebelli to the parasympathetic nuclei of the hypothalamus, specific work on the tentorium cerebelli is even more interesting when trying to attain the complete equilibration of the autonomous nervous system.

Normalizing the tentorium cerebelli might prove necessary to lift recurring restrictions of the cranial mechanism, as in the case of direct traumas that limit the lateral expansion of the cranium even after in-depth work on the nervous tissue.

Energetic work on the tentorium cerebelli is carried out using the temporal 'ear pull' procedure. Even if this procedure is similar to that of classical membranous work, the intention is different, and the aim is to restore energy in the definitive membranous structure (Fig 4.9).

For more complete work on the cranial dura mater, it is essential to consider the continuity of the endocranial membrane as well as the expansions (tentorium cerebelli and falx cerebri). The anterior and posterior aspect of the endocranial membrane can be normalized starting with a relative transversal tensing of the tentorium cerebelli.

In the posterior cranial sphere, it is possible, by varying the contact points on the auricle near the external auditory canal, to explore and normalize all of the cerebellar fossa up to the jugular foramen and even to reach the tensions affecting the foramen magnum: lightly rotating the hand in a forearm pronation movement and adding a little cubital deviation in the wrist is all that's needed. Expanding on the latter and with sufficient experience, it is possible to detect membranous tensions along the transversal aspect of the spinal dura mater located, for example, along a specific intervertebral foramen.

By inverting the contact points mentioned above for the cerebellar fossa, it is possible to explore the anterior sphere of the cranium's membranous aspect, first under the parietal bones and then in relation to the orbital plate of the frontal bone and the ethmoid bone. Through expansion, it is possible to detect tension around the anterior connections of the concave and convex borders of the tentorium cerebelli.

This work can take a long time, and requires patience and precision. During normalization, the patient can sometimes feel deep cranial tension accompanied by a burning sensation, which can be very unpleasant. Working very lightly is important for this type of work when performed on small children; another reason for using caution is that the different tissue layers of the tentorium cerebelli are not in complete continuity in very young children.

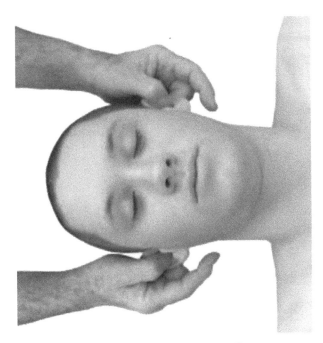

Figure 4.9. Normalization of the tentorium cerebelli.

Cranial nerve nuclei and cerebellum

The cranial nerve nuclei and the cerebellum develop from the rhombencephalon. Although anatomically and physiologically independent, these two structures are so close that they are often evaluated and normalized together. This joint work is even more useful since restrictions affecting one structure can also influence the other, their movement being inverted.

Cranial nerve nuclei

Embryological movement

The cranial nerve nuclei are located inside the neural tube at the brainstem level, and they are organized into seven columns according to their function. The fourth ventricle is formed by the forward migration of the posterior-most lateral columns in a front-facing horseshoe-shaped movement. Some of the cranial nerve nuclei allow the transmission of some of the central information that travels in the cranial nerves toward the periphery. Of course, the fourth ventricle is formed after the movement that establishes the cranial folds.

Motility movement and test

The cranial nerve nuclei migrate laterally at first before continuing in the anterior direction (horseshoe-shaped movement); it is their flexion motility movement. The global movement that establishes the nuclei enables them to pass around the fourth ventricle, thus forming it.

To evaluate the motility of the cranial nerve nuclei, the osteopath places his hands with two contact points on the occiput, on each side of the neural tube under the tentorium cerebelli. From there, he goes around the fourth ventricle in an outward movement. When this first movement is detected, the osteopath can evaluate the second (anterior) movement.

The osteopath then evaluates the cranial nerve nuclei's motility capacity (Fig. 4.10).

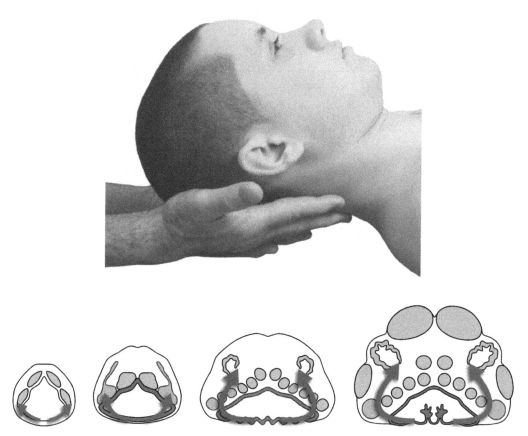

Figure 4.10. Motility of the cranial nerves nuclei.

Motility dysfunction

The cranial nerve nuclei, under a motility loss, are in an extension dysfunction state and are restricted in one or all of the components of their horseshoe-shaped movement.

Normalization

For the first part of the movement (outward expansion), normalization is usually carried out in an indirect way (accumulation).

For the second part of the movement (posteroanterior), normalization is usually carried out in the natural direction against the restriction (induction).

Before normalizing the cranial nerve nuclei, the cranial folds must be free enough to allow the circulation of information from the center toward the periphery. An isolated application of fourth ventricle techniques in their classical form can cause untimely reactions, which are understood better when considering the neurological information flow. The motility technique outlined here may look like the classical 'compression' technique for the fourth ventricle in the direction of its general movement, but its essence is completely different since it is applied on a whole other dysfunctional level. While the classical technique is based on the fluidic model (the cephalorachidian fluid), the energetic technique aims for the transmission of neurological information from the center to the periphery with specific work on the nuclei themselves. The most clinically sensitive nucleus when it comes to motility techniques is the X nucleus that transmits central parasympathetic information to the target organs and viscera of the periphery and provides a regulation effect.

Cerebellum

Embryological movement

The two cerebellar hemispheres originate from the cerebellar plates and meet along the midline, going around the fourth ventricle with a slight chronological lag.

Motility movement and test

The cerebellar peduncles, in their flexion motility movement, migrate and grow in an anteroposterior movement around the fourth ventricle at first, before moving in an inward direction.

Finally, the right and left cerebellar hemispheres move toward each other to meet along the midline.

To evaluate the cerebellum's motility, the osteopath places his hands on the occiput and under the tentorium cerebelli, on each side of the neural tube, with a slightly wider grip compared to the cranial nerve nuclei's test position described earlier. From these points, he evaluates the cerebellum's motility capacity (Fig. 4.11).

Motility dysfunction

The cerebellum, under a motility loss, is in an extension dysfunction state and is restricted in its anteroposterior movement and/or its movement toward the midline. This restriction can be unilateral or bilateral. Bilateral dysfunctions are not necessarily symmetrical.

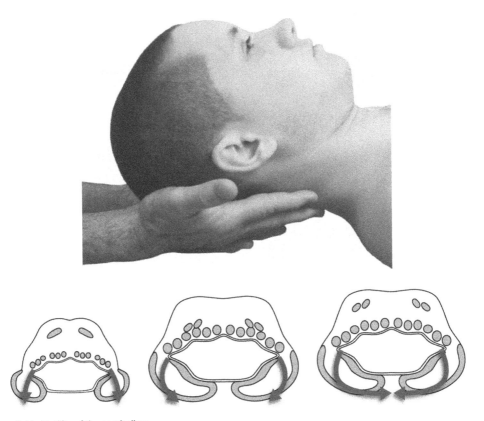

Figure 4.11. Motility of the cerebellum.

Normalization

For the first part of the movement (outward expansion), normalization is usually carried out in an indirect way (accumulation).

For the second part of the movement (posteroanterior), normalization is usually carried out in the natural direction (induction) against the restriction.

Osteopathic considerations

The cerebellum is involved in the equilibrium and regulation of fine movement. It regulates unconscious proprioception by receiving information from the homolateral hemibody. Testing and normalizing dysfunctions of the cerebellum is then especially useful when recurrent lower limb sprains occur without any real trauma, hinting at a possible proprioceptive deficit. Testing is also useful in cases of benign fine motor skills control disorders in children.

The cerebellum can also be – bilaterally – involved in equilibrium disorders like Pseudo-Ménière's disease or in the standing equilibrium and walking development of children.

By extension, dysfunctions of the cerebellum can sometimes be involved in articular disorders, such as clubfoot; clinical observations tend to confirm this.

With regard to its cognitive functions, work on the cerebellum is very useful for some learning disorders, especially language disorders – usually associated with precise work on specific zones of the cerebral hemispheres – and some attention disorders.

Finally, work on the cerebellum and the cranial nerve nuclei completes the posterior cranial sphere work.

Medulla oblongata, spinal cord, neural crest, and ganglia

To continue working on the passage of information from the autonomous nervous system to the periphery (visceral sphere), it is possible to work directly on the plexuses and viscera instead of working via the medulla oblongata, spinal cord, and neural crest. However, when faced with a chronic complaint, investigating segmental problems further by evaluating and normalizing the corresponding motility of the medullary level and/or the neural crest might prove useful. For example, for a chronic problem where the upper limbs or migraines are implicated, testing the cervicodorsal junction, since it houses the stellate ganglion, is useful; for a problem at the D10 level, dysfunctions of the adrenals would likely exist, etc. Many such examples of treatment involving the segmental innervation principle are based on the application of the core physiology that is essential to current osteopathy practice. Because it has multiple embryological relations, the remote effects of treatment of the neural crest are a realm yet to be explored.

General embryological movement of the spinal cord

The spinal cord is formed from the neural plate, which comes from the ectoderm. During its genesis, the neural plate sinks below the surface of the embryo.

The spinal cord is formed in the craniocaudal direction. It then bends along its longitudinal axis, progressively forming a tube which will become the spinal cord. This tube develops from day 22, evolving from the five superior somites and extending in the caudal direction. The movement begins with the thickening of the median part of the neural plate from back to front, causing it to wrap around itself, and finishes when the right and left folds join, sealing the posterior closing of the neural tube.

The elongation and the plication movement are evaluated using different tests.

Spinal cord
Motility movement and test

The general neural tube (spinal cord) elongation movement is cephalocaudal.

To evaluate the general motility of the spinal cord area, the osteopath runs his hand along the superior part of the vertebral column, focusing on the medullary level (inside the rachidian canal). He evaluates the neural plate's motility capacity in an upward or downward direction. This motility is expressed in two distinct flows, on the right and left. The osteopath is looking for density zones, usually symptoms of segmental spinal cord dysfunctions. When a density is found, the hand is 'stopped' in its downward movement along the vertebral column and at this level, all of the spinal cord's motility seems slowed, even if the movement is not always stopped (Fig. 4.12).

On finding one of these densities, the osteopath must stop and evaluate the plication motility of the spinal cord segment. In its flexion motility movement, as described earlier, the spinal cord segment thickens (with a slight frontward movement in the structure itself) and then rolls over on itself until the complete closure of the posterior wall.

To evaluate a spinal cord segment's plication motility, the osteopath places his hands on both sides of the appropriate medullary region. He then evaluates the spinal cord segment's motility capacity (Fig. 4.13).

Motility dysfunction

The motility loss incurred in the cephalocaudal movement of the neural plate is usually subordinate to a segmental blockage that can be evaluated with a specific test. Once this segment is normalized, the spinal cord's motility in the cephalocaudal direction should be unhindered.

The spinal cord segment, under a motility loss, is in an extension dysfunction state and is restricted in the plication movement that converts the neural plate into the neural tube. The restriction can affect one component of this plication more than others, or one side more than the other.

Normalization

Normalizing a segmental level is carried out using the indirect technique (accumulation).

When necessary, normalizing the downward positioning of the vertebral column can be achieved with natural direction techniques, complementing the segmental technique. Sometimes, this movement must be harmonized with the general movement that establishes the spinal cord, which occurs in the same direction (see Chapter 9).

Osteopathic considerations

Segmental medullary work can be useful to lift blockages of the metamere's (dermatome, myotome and/or sclerotome) general motility, or to restore the motility of the spinal nerve roots. Segmental work on the spinal cord is often

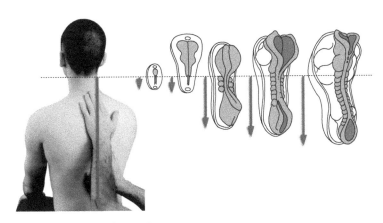

Figure 4.12. Elongation motility of the spinal cord.

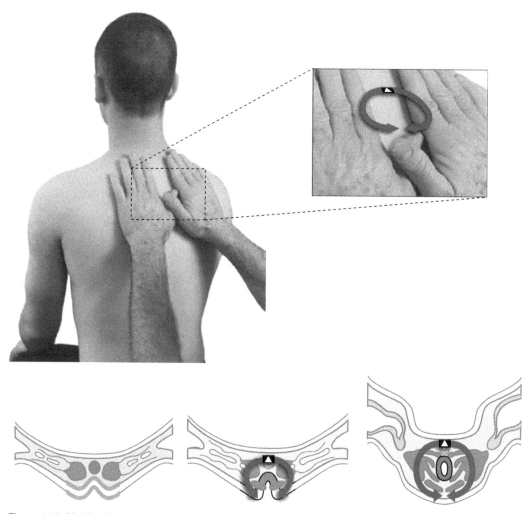

Figure 4.13. Motility of a spinal cord segment.

completed by neural crest work when a segmental level is under significant restrictions.

Segmental work on the spinal cord (and neural crest) can sometimes provide solutions for recurring or impossible-to-lift vertebral dysfunctions that resist classical osteopathic normalization techniques.

Of course, segmental work on the spinal cord is sometimes linked to specific work on the vertebra itself (see Chapter 9). Conflict between the spinal cord and the vertebra in a segment can cause chronic pain.

When applying these techniques, the experienced osteopath takes particular care to understand the context in order to prevent untimely neu-rovegetative reactions that can occur when lifting significant and/or chronic blockages in some segmental dysfunctions of the spinal cord.

Medulla oblongata

The medulla oblongata is a specific zone in the spinal cord that represents the first contact point where the neural plate becomes the tube. From this point, the neural tube is formed in both the cephalic (brain) and caudal (spinal cord) direction. This distinctive feature is worth a specific evaluation (Fig. 4.14).

Motility movement and test

To evaluate the motility of the medulla oblongata, the osteopath places his hands on both sides of the concerned medullary region, at the level of the infratentorial occiput. From there, he evaluates the medulla oblongata's motility capacity.

Motility dysfunction

The medulla oblongata, under a motility loss, is in an extension dysfunction state and is restricted in the winding movement that converts the neural plate into the neural tube. Specifically, the motility dysfunction can affect any of its embryological movement's components: the initial thickening of the anterior part, the backward movement and/or the junction of the right and left folds.

Motility loss in the medulla oblongata might sometimes be related to blockages in the superior cervical region.

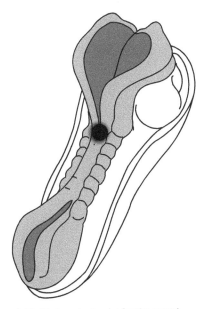

Figure 4.14. First contact point for the neural tube plication.

Normalization

Normalizing the medulla oblongata is carried out using the indirect technique (accumulation).

Neural crest and ganglia

Embryological movement

During the neural tube's development, the lateral-most parts become posterior. Cells merge at the level of the central line to form the neural crest. This new structure departs from its neural tube origin to establish itself between the ectoderm and the neural tube, becoming an independent structure. The neural crest is then divided at its central line, forming distinct right and left parts. The neural crest is the origin of the nervous ganglia that will eventually migrate in the anterior direction, passing between the somite and the neural tube toward their definitive position:

- The spinal ganglia are the first to be formed. They stay between the somite and the neural tube. The spinal ganglia transmit sensory nervous influx from the organs and viscera, the body's wall and the limbs to the spinal cord. Usually, one pair is developed per vertebral level.
- Other cells move further and are established on both sides of the developing vertebra to form the paravertebral sympathetic chain ganglia. There are two ganglia for each somite pair in the dorsal, lumbar, and sacral region. There are three in the cervical region, and only one for the coccyx. The central neurons, located in the spinal cord, are only spread in the dorsal and lumbar regions.
- At D10 level, a large number of cells migrate in the lateral and anterior direction to form the adrenal medulla.
- Going a little further, some cells form the prevertebral (pre-aortic) ganglia that wrap around a specific artery. These ganglia are related to the organization of the plexuses, as described in the following section.

• Some cells go even further, migrating along the mesenteries to form intramural ganglia in the walls of the organs and viscera. These ganglia form the second neuron of the parasympathetic system.

Motility movement and test

The neural crest's movement follows the movement of the spinal cord. When the latter is formed into the neural tube, it forms the neural crest.

In their flexion motility movement, the two parts of a neural crest are joined simultaneously with the neural tube's closure. They then detach from the neural tube in a posterior movement and split in an outward movement to form the spinal ganglia; they also subsequently form the paravertebral sympathetic chain ganglia with a posteroanterior movement. The rest of the movement is related to the establishment of the plexuses and is described later on.

To evaluate the motility of the neural crest and the ganglia, the osteopath places his hands on both sides of the neural tube and he evaluates the neural crest and ganglia's motility capacity (Fig. 4.15).

Motility dysfunction

The neural crest, under a motility loss, is in an extension dysfunction state and is restricted in one component of its movement (junction movement, posterior movement, lateral movement or anterior movement). A restriction in the anterior movement is specifically related to the ganglia.

Normalization

Normalizing the first two movements of the neural crests (junction movement and posterior

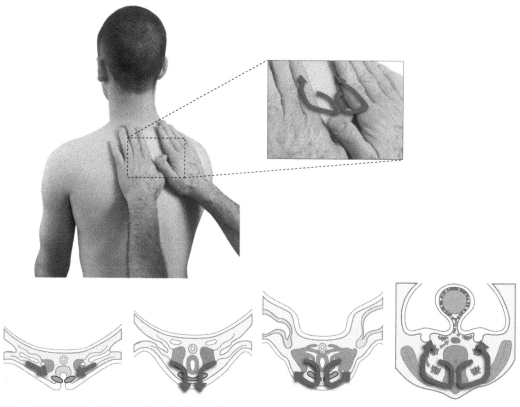

Figure 4.15. Motility of the neural crest and ganglia.

movement) is done with an indirect technique (accumulation). Normalizing the splitting movement is usually carried out using a natural direction technique (induction). Normalizing the spinal ganglia and paravertebral chain ganglia's movements is also usually carried out using an induction technique.

Osteopathic considerations

Depending on which one of the segmental levels of the neural crest is restricted, restoring the motility of the spinal and sympathetic chain ganglia will address various signs and symptoms. For example, a specific action on the D10 region will have a precise effect on the adrenal gland.

Since their anatomical distribution is extended and wide, the neural crests' motility recovery's effects can be remote and will most likely be hard to estimate precisely, even more so when these effects are combined with the effects of the other osteopathic normalizations applied over the course of the treatment.

The neural crests are responsible for the dental odontoblast's formation; embryology may explain some dental reflexologies when clinical results are confusing.

Nerve plexuses

The transmission of information from the autonomous nervous system's center to the periphery continues with work on the nerve plexuses. Nerve fibers from the cells of the neural crests form localized neurovegetative centers that move toward the heart and lungs, the intestinal tract and the renal system, the genital organs, and the skin. As explained earlier in relation to the migration of prevertebral ganglia, these nerve fibers are all related to the major circulatory axis of the thorax and abdomen. The plexuses thus provide 'food' for all tissues in the form of innervation and vascularization. According to osteopathic concepts, nerve plexuses can be linked to the classical 'Rule of the Artery'; also, in traditional Chinese medicine, blood represents energy.

Embryological movement

The movement that establishes the plexuses starts from the neural crest with the formation of ganglia and continues with the expansion of nerve fibers to the target organs. This direction of movement is frontward as well as outward. The nerve plexuses wrap around a vascular axis, and their motility movement is described as a spiral.

Motility movement and test

The flexion motility movement of the plexuses is a circular, coiled clockwise movement.

First tested is the circular inward movement originating from the periphery that is related to the penetration of information pertaining to the exterior environment. This inward movement has the same energetic circulation as its embryological counterpart, but it captures exterior energy as well as the environment's renewable energy.

The inward spiralling movement's circles decrease in circumference as they get closer to the deepest part of the plexus (its aortic junction).

This inward movement is followed by the opposite outward movement that is strictly related to the direction of embryological development. It starts with smaller circles, increasing in circumference as they move further away from the center. This outward movement is related to the person's own energy.

When entirely free, the inward and outward movements of the plexuses are each composed of seven spirals. This number of spirals was arrived at through repeated clinical experience. Because of their position, the plexuses' spirals can be linked to the chakra concept of Indian medicine and to the seven levels of consciousness. Depending on the individuals and on their functional state, the plexuses' seven spirals are not always accessible, and some restrictions are beyond the osteopathic intervention framework.

A plexus without any restriction must involve a free back-and-forth movement associated with an optimal exchange zone between the inside and outside worlds. The plexuses could be compared to antennae connected to both worlds, creating a dual interface.

Six plexuses are considered in osteopathic evaluation. The most functionally important ones are the celiac plexus and the cardiopulmonary plexus; the others are their subordinates.

To evaluate the plexuses' motility, the osteopath places his hands so that they surround the center of the evaluated plexus. He starts with the two main plexuses and moves on afterward, if needed, to the others. The exterior circumference of a plexus is proportional to its significance: the more functionally significant, the greater the circumference. Thus:

- For the **celiac plexus**, the osteopath places widespread hands on both sides of the lower part of the thorax, so that they cover a surface of which the center is the origin of the celiac plexus (just under the diaphragm, around the xiphoid process).
- For the **aorticorenal plexus**, the osteopath places his hands a little bit closer, so that they cover a surface of which the center is between the xiphoid process and the umbilicus.
- For the **superior mesenteric plexus**, the osteopath places his hands even closer together, so that they cover a surface of which the center is under the umbilicus.
- For the **inferior mesenteric plexus**, the osteopath places his hands even closer together, so that they cover a surface of which the center is between the superior mesenteric plexus and the pubic symphysis.
- For the **hypogastric plexus**, the osteopath places his hands even closer together, so that they cover a surface of which the center is above the pubic symphysis.
- For the **cardiopulmonary plexus**, the osteopath places his hands on both sides of the thorax, on the ribs, so that they cover a surface of which the center is the middle of the sternum.
- For the **hypophyseal plexus**, the osteopath places his hands so that they cover a small surface of which the center is the glabella.

The osteopath evaluates the motility capacity of the plexus in a clockwise direction, inward first and then outward. He has to be on the proper level of consciousness to precisely follow motility movement of the plexus without being distracted by the numerous surrounding structures. Evaluation starts with an active palpatory perception test and is completed by a passive palpatory perception test (Fig. 4.16).

Motility dysfunction

A plexus, under a motility loss, is in an extension dysfunction state and is restricted by either a blockage of its circular movement, a difficulty in moving onto the next spiral or total inability to complete the spiral movement. Clinically, dysfunctions affecting the two main plexuses are numerous.

Normalization

Normalization is usually carried out in the natural direction (induction) against the restriction found in the spiralled circular movement. A circular movement must be completely normalized before proceeding with the next movement.

The celiac plexus is more important than the lower plexuses since it controls the passage of the neurological information toward them. Making sure they effectively receive this necessary functional information is therefore essential before attempting localized normalizations. The celiac plexus is always evaluated and normalized first even when dysfunctions are affecting the other plexuses.

According to anatomical considerations and for the reasons mentioned above, normalizing the cardiopulmonary plexus should be carried out prior to the normalization of the hypophyseal plexus when necessary.

Osteopathic considerations

The plexuses distribute nervous influx and blood; thus, they distribute energy. They feed all

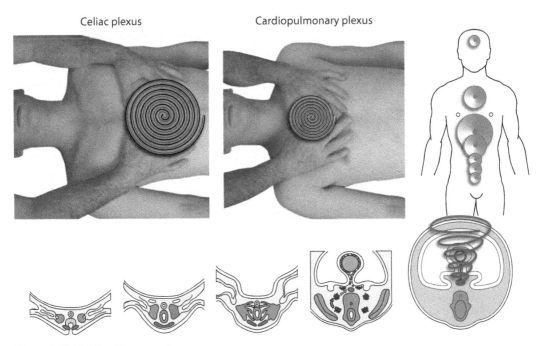

Figure 4.16. Motility of the nerve plexuses.

the structures of their segmental levels. Signs and symptoms linked to the motility dysfunction of the plexuses are therefore quite varied. Therapeutic intention is determined according to the impact on a group of organs or viscera, or, less commonly, on a specific structure. Knowing and understanding the anatomy and physiology of the autonomous nervous system is necessary in order to understand all the possible effects of normalization of the plexuses. For example, knowing that the bladder sphincter's command is under the control of the celiac plexus is essential to understanding the causes of incontinence.

Working on the plexuses can be done in the direction of the information flow, from the center to the periphery; it then follows cranial work, work on the spinal cord and/or the neural crest and work on the ganglia, and is followed by work on the organs and viscera. In some situations, the plexuses are normalized before work is carried out on the nervous system. Regulating the plexuses allows for a proper distribution of the energy that is released when working toward the periphery.

Since the plexuses are an energy exchange zone between outside and inside, both movement paths are equally important:
- The inward path of the plexus is often blocked when the organism reacts to protect itself against environmental problems. This is the most frequent type of dysfunction. The intensity of the dysfunction and also the 'height' of the restricted spiral are indicators of interest as to the state and evolution of an individual's connections with the outside world.
- The outward path of the plexus is blocked when an individual is suffering from energy distribution disorders. This dysfunction type is fortunately less frequent.

Children often suffer from plexus dysfunctions because their developing cortex lacks the consciousness and rationality to filter and be aware of relations with the outside environment. They receive, via their nerve plexuses, a lot of information from the outside world and their response is based on 'instinct'; this can sometimes explain stomach pain of an emotional origin in children, which is a common clinical occurrence.

Central nervous system: cerebral hemispheres

Embryological movement

The telencephalic vesicles, originating from the anterior brain or prosencephalon, grow in a ram's-horn-shaped winding movement. This movement is also described in classical craniosacral mechanism theory. The cerebral hemispheres' embryological growth starts with a surge behind the frontal lobe, which then rises and moves from front to back with the parietal lobe. Then, the growth energy flows to the occipital lobe, where it reverses and finally flows toward the temporal lobe, ending its journey in a spiralled outward movement.

This winding movement, wrapping around a transverse axis materialized by the foramen of Monro, is due to the very quick expansion of the hemispheres in relation to the rest of the brain. In the definitive brain, this axis lies at the level of the amygdala. With this movement, the cerebral hemispheres cover a large portion of the primitive brain (Drews 1994, p. 236).

Motility movement and test

The flexion motility movement of the cerebral hemispheres is a ram's-horn-shaped general movement (Fig. 4.17).

To evaluate the motility of the cerebral hemispheres, the osteopath places his hands on the right and left hemispheres, gradually moving to follow the motility movement. For example, he starts with his hands on the frontal lobe, feeling the surge behind it, and then feels the upward–backward movement following the ram's horn shape (Fig. 4.18).

The osteopath continues by placing his hands on each side of the vertex, then on the occipital lobe, and finally on both of the head's lateral parts to feel the surge of the temporal lobes (Fig. 4.19).

The experienced osteopath can develop a complete and inclusive hand position that allows for the complete evaluation of the motility of the hemispheres from a single position.

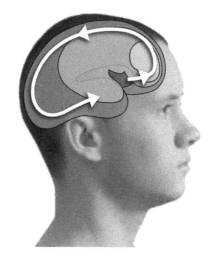

Figure 4.17. General motility of the cerebral hemispheres.

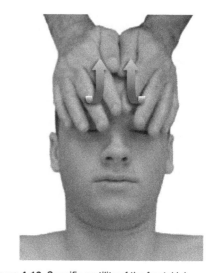

Figure 4.18. Specific motility of the frontal lobes.

Motility dysfunction

A cerebral hemisphere, under a motility loss, is in an extension dysfunction state and is restricted in one component of its ram's-horn-shaped movement.

Normalization

Normalizing the motility of the hemispheres is usually carried out in the natural direction (induction).

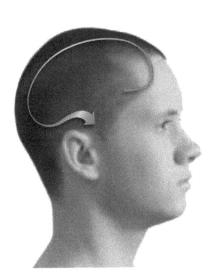
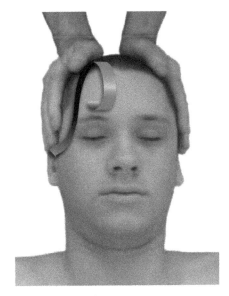

Figure 4.19. Specific motility of the temporal lobes (lateral expansion movement).

Osteopathic considerations

Signs and symptoms

Using the results of a conventional cranial evaluation, a relationship is often found between a localized increase in the osseous density of a part of the cranium and a motility dysfunction in the cerebral tissue, once again proving the primacy of the content over the container. Patients often report this density as being painful under palpation.

Many signs and symptoms can be linked to motility restrictions in parts of a cerebral hemisphere, and they can be reduced by a proper normalization. It would be illusory and simplistic, due to their extensive diversity, to try to establish an exhaustive classification of the effects of this type of intervention; furthermore, these interventions have not yet been clinically detailed. To this end, an in-depth knowledge of the anatomy and physiology of the centers of the superior central nervous system, with an emphasis on the localization of the various zones, their functions and the neurological information's path, recognizing the complexity of the anatomy and nervous system of the human being, would be useful. Brodmann's map of cerebral zones, established in the early twentieth century by the German anatomist and based on the differences in cellular architecture for the different regions of the cortex, is particularly useful to this end.

It is essential to understand the functions of the hemispheres in order to correctly analyze the motility dysfunctions identified in the evaluation process. In general, they include:

- The **occipital lobe**, which plays a significant role in extracting and analyzing physical characteristics from visual information. Thirty-two cerebral areas are linked to vision, and some of these are linked to very specific information (colors, faces, movements, etc.). The occipital lobe must answer the 'what?' (identifying the object) and the 'where?' (identifying its position) questions. It is also linked to most of the other lobes by association fibers. Information directly or indirectly related to vision uses as much as 50 per cent of the central nervous system, forming very complex circuits.

- The **parietal lobe**, which plays a part in the polysensorial somatosensory, vestibular, visual, and symbolic integration. It also has a significant function in somesthetic integration (integration of the sensorial and proprioceptive information from the periphery to the center). The parietal lobe is involved in spatial perception. The parietal eminence region, related to the fifth area of Brodmann's map (somatosen-sorial cortex), can be described as partially managing the body schema. According to the classical definition, the left parietal lobe has an analytic sequential role and the right a global synthetic role. The sensory homunculus is found at the level of the precentral gyrus. Sensory information from a hemibody is received by the contralateral hemisphere (Fig. 4.20). The parietal lobe operates closely with the other cerebral structures, which explains part of its various associated clinical symptomatology. Studying some medical syndromes gives an interesting overview of the role of the parietal lobe; it can indeed be related to repulsive apraxia, such as the rejection of food on the tongue, or to vasomotor hemisyndromes, such as shoulder–hand syndrome. Some body schema disorders related to the parietal lobe are conscious, such as losing part of the body in Alice in Wonderland syndrome or in the case of feelings of strangeness, but some others are unconscious, such as hemibody depersonalization.

- The **temporal lobe**, which is primarily associated with memory and audition, but also with language and vision. The basic function of the temporal lobe is the integration of plurimodal sensorial experiences, which gives it a significant role in general sensorial integration. The temporal lobe's development is closely related to the growth of the associative areas.

- The **frontal lobe**, which plays many roles: a specific role in language with Broca's area located in its lower posterior part, near the left coronal; a significant motor role, with the motor homunculus in the frontal part of the central sulcus, of which 80 per cent of the descending pathways are heading toward the contralateral side (Fig. 4.20). The frontal lobe houses the complex cognitive processes because it controls and organizes behavior toward a goal. It coordinates attention, memory, language, perceptions, motor skills, and limbic functions, and can be considered the center and driving force behind the modification of activities by executive functions like event anticipation, the selection of a solution to achieve an effect, planning, and the control and evaluation of the effect of an action by feedback. The frontal lobe also plays a specific role in controlling and selecting social behavior.

Reasons for consultation that might be appropriate for the use of motility techniques are sometimes complex, and many cerebral zones or structures can be involved. Here are some examples:

- The treatment of dyslexia/dysphagia may benefit from the verification of the language areas, but also the tongue's motor zone and the hypoglossal cranial nerve (XII).

- It is useful to recall the relationship between sensorial and motor homunculi, illustrated by the homunculi's presence in the central sulcus, in order to ensure effective proprioception and fine motor skills, which are related to proper motility of the hemisphere, specifically at the central sulcus, and, of course, to proper motility of the cerebellum.

- Hyperactivity and other behavioral disorders usually involve a normalization of the frontal lobe, but they can also be related to many other structures or zones of the central nervous system, depending on their particular expression.

- Medical investigation is necessary to determine epilepsy's structural or functional origin and to find effective epileptic sources, often found in the parietal or temporal lobes, but also sometimes

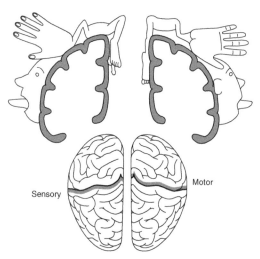

Figure 4.20. Sensory and motor homunculi.

in the frontal lobes. Functional epilepsy is, of course, more often alleviated by energetic normalization than by mechanical cranial work, and its response to treatment is better than that of structural epilepsy.

• Normalizing the lateral expansion of the temporal lobe can sometimes improve certain memory loss disorders, but these issues are very complex.

Links with cranial traumas

During particular vascular traumas of the cranium, the function that is usually linked to the traumatized zone can be hindered or completely neutralized. In some cases, cells located on the perimeter of the trauma zone are only inhibited and can profit from a normalization of their motility. This inhibition can be treated even after a very long post-traumatic time, because the function can be intact 'under' the inhibition. For cells that died during the accident leading to the trauma, there is obviously no possible action or recovery.

In the case of concussion, the aforementioned considerations are still valid, even if they have to be interpreted according to context and if, most of the time, they are related to the normalization of other central nervous system structures to allow for the best possible recovery of the patients.

Links with musculoskeletal pain

Nociceptive information from the musculoskeletal system, for example, from a peripheral articulation, the vertebral column or the pelvis, is received by the contralateral sensory homunculus. Recurring pain projections can then, in chronic or very intense cases, permeate the corresponding sensory homunculus region and cause a motility restriction in the nervous tissue that is found when evaluating the hemisphere's motility and the passage of energy at this specific location.

In these cases, since the disorder is now 'central,' localized parietal work (mechanical or motility-based) will be insufficient, if not totally ineffective, to relieve pain. This mechanism is involved in some phantom pains and is detailed below, explaining in part how to treat algoneurodystrophy

(complex regional pain syndrome) with energetic motility techniques.

This relationship was the theoretical foundation of an interesting thesis conducted by a student trained in motility techniques (Murie 2003). He led a clinical study on the effects of the nervous system's normalizations (folds, cerebellum and cerebral hemispheres) on 26 patients awaiting arthroscopic meniscal repair surgery, therefore potentially suffering from recurring knee pain. The osteopathic intervention on the nervous system was conducted just before the surgery (between 15 minutes and one hour before). A control group was formed to compare the possible effects of this intervention. Preoperative evaluations of pain (patellar ballottement test, instability, articular deficit, and quadriceps deficit) and also postoperative rehabilitation were carried out by the surgeon. Comparisons between the two groups (control and osteopathic intervention) showed that, for all the studied elements, patients that had undergone the osteopathic intervention scored higher, especially in the reduction of articular deficit (69.23 per cent improvement in the 'osteopathic' group versus 23.08 per cent for the control group), and for rehabilitation needs (26.92 per cent needed it in the osteopathic group and 46.15 per cent in the control group). These results seem significant enough to initiate studies for the validation of motility techniques and to explore their best indications.

Links with visceral nociceptive information

Nociceptive information of visceral origin is sometimes carried to the central nervous system via viscerosensory pathways. Also, clinical experience has shown that this information can sometimes be stored in an area of the first fold, homolateral and specific to the affected viscus (see the section on the first fold on p. 34 earlier in this chapter).

The organism can then manage this information in two ways:

• If visceral information toward the center stays infracortical, at the level of the first fold, the assumption is that visceral pain was not consciously felt:

- Chronic imprinting of nociceptive information can create a hemicranial restriction by reducing the amplitude of the content's motility movement, which has an impact on the same side's membranous system.
- The vertebral column and the inferior limb on the same side are frequently compressed by these membranous tensions (see Chapter 9). Secondary radiations in the lower or upper limbs of the same side, due to the effects of tension in the dura mater, can also be found.

• Nociceptive information sometimes has an impact on the infracortical tissue overlying the first fold. Usually, pain is then 'elevated' until it reaches the consciousness. The sensory homunculus described above is found in this overlying region:

- Secondary irritation of part of the sensory homunculus can cause pain in the half of the body that is contralateral to the primary visceral dysfunction. These pains are hard to objectify in their mechanical aspect and they often resist treatment, even when properly applied, since their source is not localized.
- The same homolateral dura mater restriction phenomenon described above is also found.
- The dysfunctional schema involving tension in the dura mater on the side opposed to the pain is often misunderstood, impairing the treatment's success. The interpretation grid given by embryological motility of the nervous tissue provides original and very effective clinical answers to these situations.

Complex regional pain syndrome (algoneurodystrophy)

With complex regional pain syndrome, formerly known as or algoneurodystrophy, there is a particular case for the use of nervous system motility techniques; successful results in dozens of cases amount to significant proof of the efficacy of these techniques.

For many patients, the emergence of symptoms of complex regional pain syndrome is explained by an intense stress, usually related to a certain degree of pre-existing hypersympatheticotonia causing the inability, in the affected patients, to autoregulate themselves and eliminate nociceptive information. The majority of the affected subjects therefore show anxious characteristics.

The effects of stress, as previously explained, have an impact on the first fold, but a very intense stress 'overflows' onto the level of the third fold as well. Furthermore, somatic pain in the superior or inferior limbs is processed by the contralateral homunculus and by the homolateral cerebellum.

These motility dysfunctions of the central nervous system, together with their great intensity, indicate a significant autonomous nervous system disorder. The result is chronic pain in the affected limb(s), even if purely somatic components were declining before the halt in recovery and the development of the algoneurodystrophy. The regular recovery process is then superseded by various symptoms: intense pain, alterations in the skin or neurovegetative localized disorders often leading to demineralization of the bones. This pain and functional loss are chronic and disabling and they find little or no solution in known therapies.

A proper energetic motility treatment, when it is effective, can resolve most of the problems caused by complex regional pain syndromes in a shorter time than other known treatments.

Scientific developments concluding that complex regional pain syndrome is a central nervous system disorder rather than a localized effect of the autonomous nervous system (Jänig and Baron 2003, Moseley and Flor 2012) tend to confirm the usefulness of motility treatment. The effectiveness of treatment in which the patient watches and moves his or her healthy limb in front of a mirror also confirms the nervous system's causality in these pathologies: indeed, the reversed image sends a message to the brain, telling it the affected limb can exist and move without pain. This 'lie' contributed to improvement and recovery in numerous cases of complex regional pain syndrome (Tichelaara et al. 2007, Ramachandran and Rogers-Ramachandran 1996).

Further considerations

The evaluations and normalizations of many central nervous system structures are presented in this chapter. These examples provide an overview of the possibilities of this type of intervention. Applying these principles to the embryological movements of other structures is likely to open up new fields of intervention and treatment.

References

Botez M I, Lalonde R and Botez-Marquard T (1996) Le cervelet: Comportement moteur et non-moteur, in De Botez M I (ed) Neuropsychologie clinique et neurologie du comportement, 2ème édition. Montréal: Les Presses de l'Université de Montréal/ Editions Masson.

Cochard L R (2015) Atlas d'embryologie humaine de Netter Trans. Stéphane Louryan. De Boeck.

Drews U (1994) Atlas de poche d'embryologie. Broché Flammarion Médecine-Sciences.

Jänig W and Baron R (2003) Complex regional pain syndrome: mystery explained? Lancet Neurol 2 (11) November 687–697.

Juster R-P, McEwen B S and Lupien S J (2010) Allostatic load biomarkers of chronic stress and impact on health and cognition. Neuroscience and Biobehavioral Reviews 35 (1) September 2–16.

Liem T (2010) Ostéopathie crânienne: manuel pratique. Paris: Maloine.

Molinari M, Leggio M G and Silveri M (1997) Verbal fluency and agrammatism, in Schmahmann J D (ed) The cerebellum and cognition. San Diego: Academic Press.

Moseley G L and Flor H (2012) Targeting cortical representations in the treatment of chronic pain: a review. Neurorehabilitation & Neural Repair 26 (6) July–August 646–652.

Murie Y (2003) Arthroscopie du genou et ostéopathie: influence de l'harmonisation de certains paramètres des systèmes nerveux central et autonome, en pré-opératoire Diplôme en ostéopathie, Institut Supérieur d'Ostéopathie.

Ramachandran V S and Rogers-Ramachandran D (1996) Synaesthesia in phantom limbs induced with mirrors. Proceedings: Biological Sciences 263 (1369) April 377–386.

Tichelaar Y I, Geertzen J H, Keizer D and Van Wilgen C P (2007) Mirror box therapy added to cognitive behavioural therapy in three chronic complex regional pain syndrome type I patients: a pilot study. International Journal of Rehabilitation Research 30 (2) June 181–188.

Chapter 5

Psychoneuroimmune-Endocrine System

Endocrine System

Summary

This first section focuses on the endocrine part of the psychoneuroimmune-endocrine system. After some general considerations, the hypophysis, pineal gland, and thyroid will be described. The other glands are described elsewhere in this book. The distinctive features of the endocrine system are usually investigated after dysfunctions of the nervous system have been normalized, since the former partially depends on the latter.

The endocrine system is one of the main regulation systems and is part of the subtle and complex integrated system known as the psychoneuroimmune-endocrine system, which is influenced by many elements ranging from the chemical, physical, and psychological equilibriums to external factors like temperature or light.

The endocrine system is made up of a combination of hormone-producing glands led by the hypothalamic–pituitary axis. The pineal gland is found in the cranium, while the other glands are located in the thorax (thyroid and parathyroid), the abdomen (abdominal, adrenal, and pancreas) or the pelvis (testicles and ovaries). Many other structures produce hormones: the walls of the stomach, duodenum, small intestine, kidneys, and heart, and also the thymus. During pregnancy, the placenta is also a significant source of hormones (Marieb 2005).

The endocrine system plays roles in energetic equilibrium by regulating the internal environment and managing cellular activity, in development and growth, in reaction to the environment (infections, stress, hunger, hemorrhage, temperature regulation, etc.) and in reproductive processes.

Unlike information originating from the nervous system, hormones circulate through blood to reach their target tissue. Endocrine messages can then take quite some time to be received. However, their effects are usually long-lasting. The endocrine system mostly works with feedback loops between production centers, inhibiting hormones, and target organs.

This chapter covers the hypophysis, pineal gland, and thyroid. The adrenal glands are covered in Chapter 4 on the nervous system, via their link with the neural crests at the D10 level. The endocrine pancreas is covered, along with its exocrine counterpart, in Chapter 7, and gonads are covered in Chapter 8.

Hypophysis

The hypophysis can be divided into two distinct parts:
- The posterior hypophysis comes from the diencephalon (neurological origin); it releases two types of hormones, produced by the hypothalamus: oxytocin and the antidiuretic hormone (ADH).
- The anterior hypophysis develops from Rathke's pouch; stimulated by hormones released by the hypothalamus, the anterior hypophysis secretes and releases six hormones: growth hormone (GH), prolactin (PRL), follicle-stimulating hormone (FSH), luteinizing hormone (LH), thyrotropin (TSH), and adrenocorticotropic hormone – also known as corticotropin – (ACTH).

The hypophysis has an effect on almost all the functions of the endocrine system.

Embryological movement

The posterior part of the movement of the hypophysis is downward from the hypothalamus, slightly in front of the anterior wall of the first fold, and because of this the movement of the neurohypophysis is partially linked to the flexion capacity of the first fold.

The anterior part of the movement of the hypophysis is upward through the sphenoid bone between the presphenoid and postsphenoid, its axis following the vomer. The two parts merge to form the definitive hypophysis.

Motility movement and test

The normal motility movement of the posterior part of the hypophysis is a downward movement from the hypothalamus, and that of the anterior part is an upward movement through the sphenoid.

To evaluate the motility of both parts, the osteopath places one hand on the vertex toward the sella turcica and the other inside the mouth or under the chin, toward the sella turcica. He checks if both energetic movements merge at the sella turcica, which would indicate a normal motility of both parts of the hypophysis (Fig. 5.1).

Restrictions in the downward movement of the posterior hypophysis can also be found when testing the first fold's upward movement; they will be revealed to the osteopath if he focuses on the movements permitted in the dense tissue of the anterior wall. Even if restrictions can be found during the first fold's movement, clinical observations have not shown that restrictions in the movement of the posterior hypophysis can hinder it.

Motility dysfunction

The hypophysis, under a motility loss, is in an extension dysfunction state and is restricted in one or both of the movements allowing its two parts to merge at the sella turcica.

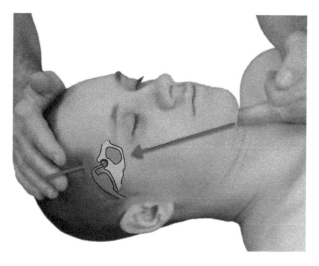

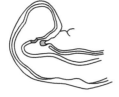 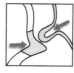 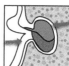

Figure 5.1. Motility of the hypophysis.

Normalization

Normalizing the motility of the hypophysis is usually carried out in the natural direction (induction), and it must restore synchronism between the two movements.

Osteopathic considerations

Hypophysis dysfunctions can be linked to various functions, according to indicators given as the reason for consultation: for example, ovarian cycle irregularity, growth problems in children, neuroendocrine system-related mood disorders, etc. Listing all of these would take too long and the reader should refer to the works referenced in this chapter for further information.

Pineal gland (epiphysis cerebri)

The pineal gland clings to the roof of the third ventricle in the diencephalon. Because it produces melatonin, mostly during the night, it is considered as the superior center controlling the organism's active or resting state according to the light available. To this end, the pineal gland receives retinal information, which passes through sympathetic pathways via the hypothalamus and the superior cervical ganglion before reaching the gland using secondary arteries. Although the pineal gland's functions are not yet entirely understood, it could be implicated in the ageing process (Marieb 2005).

Embryological movement

Initially located in the superior part of the diencephalon, in the same frontal plane as the hypophysis (in the inferior part), the pineal gland goes backward by 90 degrees when establishing itself. This movement is mostly due to the posterior rotation of the diencephalon in its definitive establishing movement. The pineal gland, with this movement, seems to go 'around' the superior part of the thalamus, stopping at the posterior part of the corpus callosum.

Motility movement and test

The 90 degrees backward movement is the normal motility movement of the pineal gland.

To evaluate the pineal gland's motility, the osteopath places one hand on the sagittal suture and, finding the proper depth level, he tests the pineal gland's motility capacity (Fig. 5.2).

Motility dysfunction

The pineal gland, under a motility loss, is in an extension dysfunction state and is restricted in its backward movement.

Normalization

Normalizing the pineal gland's motility is usually carried out in the natural direction (induction).

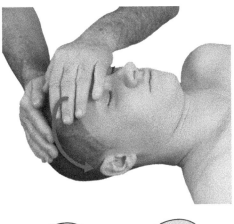

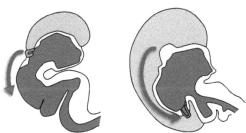

Figure 5.2. Motility of the pineal gland.

Osteopathic considerations

Because of its role in the circadian rhythm, normalizing the pineal gland gives impressive results for adaptation disorders related to time-zone changes, but it is also recommended for all other day or night rhythm disorder types.

Since the production of melatonin is linked to vitiligo, normalizing the pineal gland could be recommended for this type of problem.

Thyroid

The thyroid secretes thyroxine (T4) and triiodothyronine (T3) which are the main metabolism stimulation hormones. The thyroid hormones both contain iodine.

The parafollicular cells of the thyroid secrete calcitonin, which reduces blood calcium. They have effects on the basal metabolism (temperature regulation), on blood pressure control, on the growth and development of tissues, especially osseous and nervous tissues, and they are essential to reproductive functions (Marieb 2005). Parathyroid glands secrete the parathyroid hormone (PTH), which increases blood calcium.

Embryological movement

The thyroid appears as a bud located on the posterior third of the tongue, and is divided into two parts during its downward movement toward its definitive position, forming the bilobed thyroid.

Motility movement and test

The thyroid's normal motility movement is a downward movement followed by a splitting movement.

To evaluate the thyroid's motility, the osteopath places his hands on the anterior part of the neck and tests the thyroid's motility capacity (Fig. 5.3).

Motility dysfunction

The thyroid, under a motility loss, is in an extension dysfunction state and is restricted in its downward and/or splitting movement.

Normalization

Normalizing the thyroid's motility is usually carried out in the natural direction (induction).

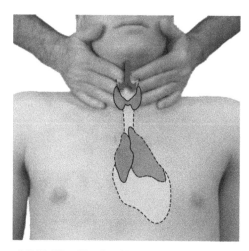
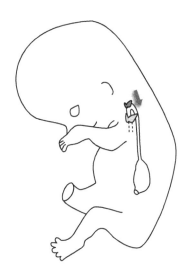

Figure 5.3. Motility of the thyroid.

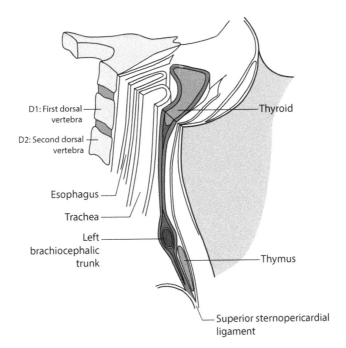

D1: First dorsal vertebra

D2: Second dorsal vertebra

Esophagus

Trachea

Left brachiocephalic trunk

Thyroid

Thymus

Superior sternopericardial ligament

Figure 5.4. Fascia linking the thyroid to the pericardium.

Osteopathic considerations

The fascia linking the thyroid to the pericardium wraps around the posterior wall of the thymus and includes the left brachiocephalic trunk, which drains all of the body's lymph except for the head and upper right limb (they use the thoracic duct). This fascia is related to the general lymphatic drainage of the body (and especially of the thyroid).

This fascia is also a link between the thoracic plication and the thymus, which is one of the important components of the immune system, especially in children (Fig. 5.4).

Immune system

Summary

This section focuses on the immune function of the psychoneuroimmune-endocrine system. Theoretical considerations will be followed by descriptions of the thymus and the spleen. The other components of the immune system are covered elsewhere in this book.

The distinctive features of the immune system are usually investigated after the normalization of dysfunctions of the nervous system since the former partially depend on the latter.

The immune system distinguishes the cells that make up your body (self) and will try to get rid of anything that does not belong in the body (non-self). Indeed, it continuously forms lymphocytes, able and responsible for the recognition of self-antigens to which it does not react (immune tolerance mechanism). This capacity for self-recognition is what allows for the recognition of the non-self-antigens, usually of a microbial origin, that the immune system fights in order to maintain the organism's integrity (Abbas & Lichtman 2009).

An immune system dysfunction (immunodeficiency) increases the possibility of infections, the incidence rate of some cancers, and can also cause latent infections to activate, like the Epstein–Barr virus, tuberculosis or cytomegalovirus (Abbas & Lichtman 2009).

An altered self-recognition mechanism can lead to autoimmune diseases caused by improper self-antigen response. Those diseases, often triggered by environmental factors, affect 1 to 2 per cent of the population in developed countries. They are often activated by a primary infection for which the immune response was abnormal (Abbas & Lichtman 2009).

The line between self and non-self is sometimes blurred, as highlighted, for example, in research on microchimerism, which is the transfer of fetal cells to the mother that induces a usually beneficial immune system stimulation in her organism (Boyon & Vinatier 2011).

The functions of the immune system are greatly influenced by the psychological and emotional general state and also by the state of the autonomous nervous system, the endocrine system, and many components of the central nervous system. The combination of all these components forms an integrated system – the psychoneuroimmune-endocrine system. Techniques related to the autonomous and central nervous systems are then useful for the regulation of the functions of the immune system (see Chapter 5). In a macroscopic way, motility techniques can greatly influence the organs of the immune system, such as the upper respiratory tracts (Waldeyer's tonsillar ring), the thymus, the spleen and the Peyer patches of the small intestine (their normalization is described in Chapter 7).

Thymus

The thymus ensures immunity over the course of a person's lifespan, although it is less active in adults than in children. It is rather voluminous and sits, along with the heart, in the mediastinal cavity. It is one of the endocrine system's glands since it secretes thymosin, which programs T-lymphocytes.

Embryological movement

The thymus develops from two lateral thymic buds that descend down the throat in an inward movement, merging at the central line to form one thymus. The merging point is called the thymic 'V.'

Motility movement and test

The normal motility movement of the two thymic buds is a downward, slightly inward movement.

To evaluate the motility of the thymus, the osteopath places his hands on the anterior part of the neck and tests the motility capacity of the thymus (Fig. 5.5).

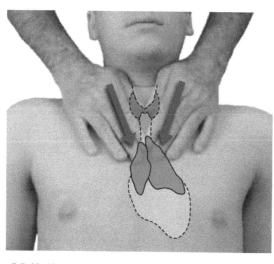
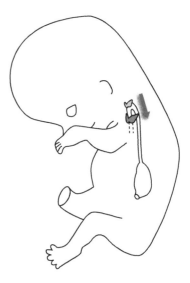

Figure 5.5. Motility of the thymus.

Motility dysfunction

The thymus, under a motility loss, is in an extension dysfunction state and is restricted in the downward or merging movements of its two buds.

Normalization

Normalizing the motility of the thymus is usually carried out in the natural direction (induction).

Osteopathic considerations

The motility of the fascia linking the thyroid to the pericardium can be disrupted by an intense postvaccinal reaction, which affects the thymus (see Fig. 5.4). The overstimulated fascia seems to react by showing a secondary inhibition, of which the possible effects were described above (see the section on Thyroid).

Spleen

The spleen, a lymphoid organ, plays a significant role in immunity since it houses a large number of lymphocytes, phagocytes, and antibodies. The spleen also plays a role in the maturation and elimination of red blood cells, but its other functions are yet to be clearly demonstrated.

Embryological movement

The spleen develops from the mesoderm and appears directly in the posterior mesogastrium, behind the stomach. The gastrosplenic ligament's development is therefore easy to understand. The spleen then moves slightly to the left, into the left hypochondrium.

Motility movement and test

The spleen's normal motility movement is a translation to the left. It seems to complete the movement of the endocrine pancreas and is located on the same plane. It can be clinically useful to verify the synchronism between these two organs.

To evaluate the spleen's motility, the osteopath stands to the right of the subject. He places his right hand, with his left hand directly over it, on the left rib cage and tests the spleen's motility capacity. He should be able to feel the surge originating from the establishing movement.

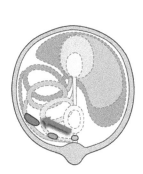

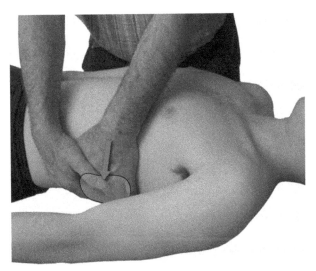

Figure 5.6. Motility of the spleen.

If the osteopath wants to verify the synchronism of the spleen and pancreas, he places one hand on the spleen and the other on the pancreas (Fig. 5.6).

Motility dysfunction

The spleen, under a motility loss, is in an extension dysfunction state and is restricted in its left translation movement. The osteopath cannot feel its lateral surge against the rib cage.

Normalization

Normalizing the spleen is usually carried out with the indirect technique (accumulation). The spleen can sometimes show energy deficiency dysfunctions.

When focusing on synchronism between the spleen and the mesogastrium and/or the endocrine pancreas, the accumulation normalization of the spleen is combined with the induction normalizations of these structures.

Links with traditional Chinese medicine

When linked to an emotion, spleen dysfunctions are linked to melancholy. When linked to a climatic element, the spleen is linked to humidity. With the liver, the spleen's proper motility is essential for the passage of the kidney's energy that provides the body with vital energy.

Osteopathic considerations

In addition to the classical osteopathic considerations relating to the spleen, an extension motility dysfunction of the spleen can be related to dysfunctions of the mesogastrium that can sometimes hinder the correct movement of the adjacent stomach.

References

Abbas A K and Lichtman A H (2009) Les bases de l'immunologie fondamentale et clinique. Paris: Elsevier Masson.

Boyon C and Vinatier D (2011) Microchimérisme foetal: soi et nonsoi, finalement qui sommes-nous? Journal de Gynécologie Obstétrique et Biologie de la Reproduction 40 (5) September 387–398.

Marieb E N (2005) Anatomie et physiologie humaines. Montréal: Editions du renouveau pédagogique.

Chapter 6

Cardiopulmonary System

Summary

This chapter focuses on two complementary systems located in the thorax and the cardiac and pulmonary systems. The cardiac system includes not only the heart itself, but also its pericardial serous and fibrous envelopes. The pleuropulmonary system includes the pulmonary parenchyma and the pleurae. The significance of dysfunctions found in these systems for clinical practice and their impact are discussed, and also tests and normalization techniques. The pericardium is a structure often found to be dysfunctional and must be considered early in clinical interventions, often at the same time as the thoracic plication.

Although they are located in the same cavity, the heart, lungs, and their envelopes do not share the same types of dysfunction, and the impact of their dysfunctions is also very different. However, if one thoracic structure is restricted in its movement, it can often significantly influence the others, resulting in compensations in the whole thorax.

The establishment of the heart and its protective envelopes begins early in the development of the embryo, in the same embryological movement as the thoracic plication. Work on the frequently dysfunctional pericardial structures is often essential for a complete normalization of this plication, especially on the fibrous pericardium, since it is closely related to the diaphragmatic mechanism, in which it regulates part of the movement of the phrenic center. Since it is the anchoring point for all the pericardial ligaments, normalizing the fibrous pericardium will impact its anchors (upper dorsal vertebrae and sternum) and, following fascial continuity, the base of the cranium. Work on the heart, the pericardia and the ligament structures has significant mechanical, emotional, and general effects.

Lungs should be treated differently according to which structure (the parenchyma, the visceral pleura or the parietal pleura) is in a dysfunctional state. The difference between a unilateral dysfunction and a dysfunction involving both lungs should be considered during the clinical evaluation.

Embryological generalities

Formation of the container of the thorax is dependent on the movement of the thoracic fold as described in Chapter 3; this movement brings the septum transversum to the diaphragm's location in the definitive body. Formation of the walls of the thoracic container is achieved with the establishment of the lateral folds. As for the abdomen, but unlike the cranium, the establishment of the thoracic container happens before its contents are established.

Not all elements of the contents of the thorax develop from the same embryological origin. The heart and outflow tracts are from the splanchnopleuric region mesoblast. The pulmonary system and the trachea develop from the anterior intestine, and they are of the same embryological origin as the esophagus.

Heart, and serous and fibrous pericardia

There is no further need to explain the heart's functional role. The osteopath must still keep it in mind, ensuring optimal operation and respecting the differences between function and structure. Fortunately, most of the work will be related to the fibrous pericardium and its ligaments, and not the heart itself; the pericardial ligaments and the pericardium's dual layer do a great job of protecting the heart, effectively bearing tensions, shocks, and traumas (especially high-speed ones), occasionally forcing a postural adaptation to provide the best possible conditions for the functionality of the cardiac muscle. In order to achieve lasting results when normalizing dysfunctions of the cardiopulmonary system, it is essential to understand both the causes of the dysfunctions and the hierarchy of functions in the body.

Embryological movement

As blood distribution is essential for the growth of the embryo's tissues, the heart is the first functional organ, operating as soon as it is formed. The circulatory system's precursors start working at day 22 (heart) and day 24 (general blood circulation). The primary role of the heart can be related to A. T. Still's famous saying: 'The rule of the artery is supreme.'

At the end of the third week, the cardiac progenitor cells, or primary heart tubes, are located in the superior part of the embryo, over the anterior neuropore – therefore, over what will become the head. They then become, around the fourth week, two endocardial tubes that will merge, forming

one embryonic primitive cardiac tube. Between the fifth and eighth weeks, the cardiac tube goes through many iterations (looping, remodeling, realignment, and septation), which form its definitive aspect and establish the four heart chambers.

Overall, the heart performs three different movements during the process of establishment.

As described in Chapter 3, the first movement occurs during the thoracic folding: the cardiac progenitor cells rotate by 180 degrees and descend, passing in front of the cervical and dorsal vertebrae. The primitive heart is established just above the septum transversum. The fibrous pericardium follows the heart in this first movement (Fig. 6.1A).

With the heart established in the thorax in this way, the precursors of the ventricles are initially located above the precursors of the atria. The heart then grows quickly and elongates. It folds over on itself and rotates by 180 degrees again, bringing the atria over the ventricles. During this time, intense reworking allows for the initial establishment of the main veins and arteries; they will only become definitive at birth. The serous pericardium follows the heart in this second movement (Fig. 6.1B).

Finally, to establish the aorta and pulmonary trunk, the heart twists on itself. Now in its definitive form, the heart's superior part, with the large vessels, tilts to the right, and the heart's apex is to the left. The 'draining' of the heart, during

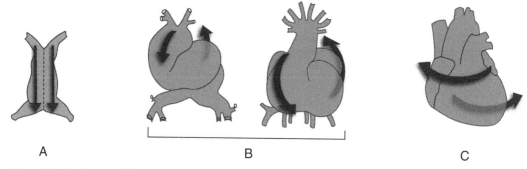

A   B   C

Figure 6.1. The three establishing movements of the heart.
A : Descent and 180-degree rotation of the cardiac progenitor cells.
B : Growth and second 180-degree rotation of the heart.
C : Definitive establishment of the heart's apex and large vessels.

contraction, will be eased by this twisted structure. As in the second movement, the serous pericardium follows the heart in this torsion movement (Fig. 6.1C).

Motility movement and test

Three distinct movements are evaluated for the heart and the serous and fibrous pericardia.

The first movement is the downward movement, relating to the heart and both the pericardia, that occurs at the same time as the beginning of the thoracic plication. This descending movement is reflected in the definitive human body by the fascia which stretch between the thyroid and pericardium; the downward movement of the thoracic plication is reflected in the anterior part of the mediastinum. Restrictions in this movement greatly affect the fibrous pericardium and, since the latter has to protect the heart, restrictions are extremely common. These restrictions are obviously frequently associated with deficiencies in the thoracic plication's movement and often both must be normalized simultaneously for effective results (Fig. 6.2).

The second and third movements relate only to the heart and the serous pericardium.

The second movement is the 360-degree rotation movement composed of the two successive 180-degree rotations the heart makes while establishing itself definitively. Thus, the heart's motility is illustrated by a constant and perpetual rotation on itself. Variations in the flexion's amplitude give the palpatory impression of a camshaft rotation movement, the spikes being caused by the flexion movements.

The heart is the only organ of which the motility is a perpetual movement. Motility disorders are fortunately rare, since they usually indicate problems within the structure of the heart. Restrictions of this order require immediate medical attention.

To properly evaluate this perpetual rotation movement, the oblique axis of the heart, caused by the torsion movement (see third movement), must be taken into account. The direction of the oblique axis is from the upper left (global direction of the left shoulder) to the lower right (global direction of the right ilium).

To evaluate the heart's motility around its oblique axis, the osteopath places his hands on the

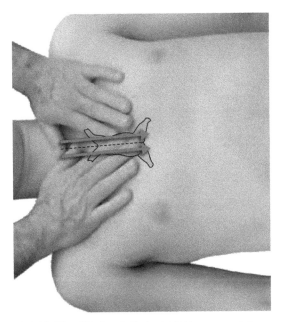

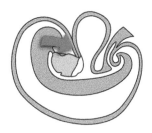

Figure 6.2. Motility of the heart's first establishing movement.

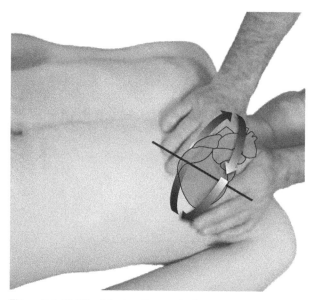

Figure 6.3. Motility of the heart's perpetual movement.

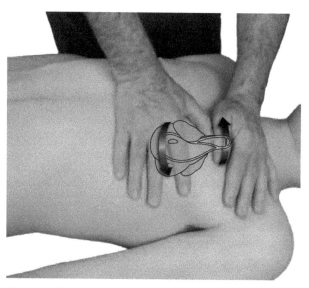

Figure 6.4. Motility of the establishing movement of the heart's apex and large vessels.

thorax at the level of the heart and evaluates its perpetual rotation motility capacity around the oblique axis (Fig. 6.3).

The third movement is the self-twisting movement that establishes the outflow tracts and the heart's apex. The osteopath places his hands over and under the oblique axis and evaluates the motility movement's capacity to bring, under the axis, the heart's tip to the left, and over the axis, the large vessels to the right. As with the second movement, dysfunctions are quite rare. If they do occur, they can be related to a structural problem in the heart or to significant digestive disorders (for a full explanation see Osteopathic considerations in the Stomach section in Chapter 7) (Fig. 6.4).

Motility dysfunction

The fibrous pericardium, under a motility loss, is restricted in its downward movement represented by the fascia stretched between the thyroid and pericardium. These dysfunctions are common.

The heart and the serous perdicardium, under a motility loss, are either:

• restricted in their perpetual rotation motility; or
• restricted in their motility around the oblique axis representing the establishment of the outflow tracts to the right and the heart's apex to the left.

These dysfunctions are rare.

Normalization

Normalizing the fibrous pericardium's motility is carried out in the natural direction (induction).

When dysfunctions are found, normalizing the heart and the serous pericardium is also usually carried out in the natural direction.

Links with traditional Chinese medicine

When associated with an emotion, dysfunctions of the heart are linked to an excess of joy.

Osteopathic considerations

Energy excess of the thorax

The most difficult normalization seems to be for the thorax under an energy-excess dysfunction. The significant density encountered in the thorax often means it is resistant to conventional techniques. In the majority of cases, a dysfunction in the establishing movement of the thoracic plication is found, along with specific dysfunctions relating to the establishment of the fibrous pericardium. A thorax in an energy-excess state are sometimes associated with a cardiopulmonary plexus dysfunction, which makes the situation even more complex by reducing vascular and nervous input to the thoracic tissues. As mentioned in Chapter 3, thoraxes in an energy-excess state are also associated with celiac plexus dysfunctions; the second movement of the thoracic plication is thus especially hindered.

When the whole thoracic region is affected, its motility is generally hindered, especially if the restrictions have been there for a long time and have become chronic. As collateral victims of the container's dysfunctions, the lungs are often affected by a bilateral extension dysfunction. These situations inevitably cause a decline in the amplitude of diaphragmatic inspiration, associated with a deficiency in the descending movement of the phrenic center, dysfunctions of the cervicodorsal junction and/or occiput-atlas-axis (OAA) junction, and too many demands on the cranial base from the tissular continuity of the deep fasciae. This situation can become more complicated if a dysfunction of the esophagus is also present or if the esophagus is affected by anxiety or environmental dysfunctions.

Adaptive postural changes are, in these cases, often observed. The musculoskeletal system moves in to protect both the heart and respiratory system by bringing the pericardial ligament's insertions closer to allow for the deepest possible inspiration. The typical posture of a person affected by energy excess of the thorax is characterized by a rigid thorax with a reduced thoracic expansion and a flat surface between the shoulder blades despite a globally enhanced kyphosis. The cervicodorsal junction seems 'broken,' with the presence of a Dowager's hump, or at least of a localized cellulalgia. The head is protracted, putting the infra-occipital region under a significant mechanical tension and weakening it.

Symptoms in this situation might be head pain (headaches and migraines), or vertebral or upper limb pain, due to the compression adaptation incurred for the relief of thoracic tensions.

The reasons for consultation are various but the common characteristic is chronicity and resistance to local techniques in treatment. Symptoms can also be related to the visceral sphere, because of the lack of general stimulation of the abdomen's viscera by the diaphragm.

Causes of an energy-excess dysfunction of the thorax are often either emotional or associated with trauma; they could also come from an excessive stress that was impossible to manage in real time or to dissipate early after the disruptive events. Rapid normalization cannot be expected, and the golden rule is to respect the tissues. As Sutherland wisely said: 'For healthy tissues, quick response. For damaged tissues, slow response.'

Patients must be advised of the possible effects of normalization of significant thoracic dysfunctions, such as intense emotional states or fatigue persisting for a few days following treatment. Patients should also be aware that when tissues agree to gain back normal movement after undergoing intense emotional traumas, the somatization process, which was useful and essential at first, heals by allowing the consciousness to 'remember.' The healing process can also proceed without consciousness, which is totally acceptable in most cases. Unfortunately, normalizing some dysfunctions will be impossible due to the initial traumas being too intense or significant, and to the protection mechanisms being too deeply rooted.

Due to the extremely high rate of occurrence and its significant impact, particular care is required to detect and normalize this type of dysfunctional schema. Energetic motility techniques provide very effective methods, especially when paired with work on the central nervous system.

Links with the health of the heart and vascular system

During the diaphragm's inspiration movement, the heart tends toward verticality without descending as low as the phrenic center, since the fibrous pericardium partially rotates on itself and this posterior rotation prevents an excessive

tension in the large vessels. A differential movement occurs between the serous and fibrous pericardia, made possible by the sliding surface created between both membranes.

This differential movement has a likely mechanical influence on the coronary sinus since the latter is located just under the fold of the pericardia in the posterior part of the heart.

The coronary sinus is very important for cardiac function and for maintaining blood volume because of its 'pressure pump' role, causing the distension of the walls of the right atrium where atrial-natriuretic-factor or ANF-producing glands (the atrial myocytes) are located. ANF is a diuretic substance that reinforces the heart muscle's power without increasing its rhythm. Its production is enabled by distension of the walls of the right atrium, where the coronary sinus is located.

The coronary sinus, being strategically located at the fold of the pericardia, benefits from a mechanical stimulation during deep inhalation. A simple and cost-free way to prevent heart disease is by giving freedom to the movement of the diaphragm and by making a habit of inhaling deeply. The ability to inhale deeply is relevant to osteopathy, which sees it as a wide-ranging and essential preventive method (Figs. 6.5 and 6.6).

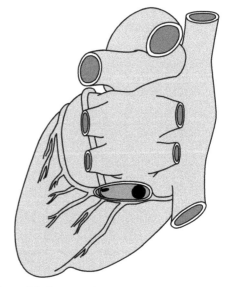

Figure 6.5. Coronary sinus.

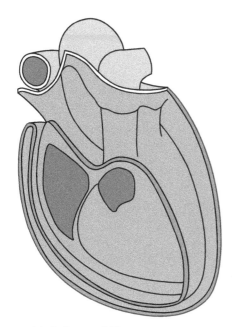

Figure 6.6. Peritoneum fold.

Pulmonary system

The lungs are part of the lower respiratory tract, which extends from the trachea to the alveoli, while the upper respiratory tract extends from the mouth to the larynx–pharynx region. The lungs' main function is of course gas exchange; they provide an oxygen supply to the body and, therefore, energy. They also act as an exit path for the body's waste, not just for carbon dioxide but also for various toxins. They help regulate the acid-base balance and play a role in blood filtration (filtration of small clots). Before reaching the lungs, air is usually warmed up, humidified, and purified by the mucosal lining of the respiratory tract.

The right lung has three lobes while the left has only two since the size of the left lung is restricted by the heart. Pulmonary fissures separate the lobes, allowing for their relative movement.

The pleurae surround the pulmonary parenchyma in the same way as the peritoneum surrounds viscera and organs. They facilitate sliding. The visceral pleura, or serous pleura, surrounds the lungs whereas the parietal pleura lines the thoracic cavity (mostly ribs and diaphragm). Between the two pleurae, a few milliliters of serous fluid are found in the pleural cavity.

The pleurae and lungs are prompted by around 24,000 breaths a day. This very high number of small, repeated movements, along with the outstanding mechanical capacity of the multi-articulated thorax to adapt, may explain the long delay between the beginning of an osteopathic dysfunction and the emergence of signs and symptoms.

Embryological movement

Lungs originate from a bud located at the anterior part of the anterior intestine, called the respiratory diverticulum. During its development, this bud will undergo many modifications. The first one is its division into two lungs, happening between the 26th and 28th day. The lungs progressively expand into 16 branching generations, resulting in the formation of the terminal bronchioles between the sixth and 16th week. Each terminal bronchiole is then divided into two or more respiratory bronchioles. Vascularization of the lungs occurs between the 16th and 28th week. From the 28th week to the 36th, the primitive alveoli appear, and they will finish their development throughout the rest of childhood. From the 36th week, the lungs are considered to be developed enough to allow the child to breathe without assistance after birth.

For the thorax, as the container is established before its contents, the parietal pleura is established at the same time as the lateral plication movement, slightly before the visceral pleura. The lungs then grow inside the pleural cavities like a fist sinking into a balloon. Because of their growth, the visceral pleura is pressed against them, while the parietal pleura lines the internal wall of the thorax, the diaphragm and the mediastinum. In the definitive thorax, the space between the two pleurae becomes virtual and houses a small quantity of serous fluid that helps reduce the friction between the two layers during breathing.

The definitive development of the container is completed by the growth of the ribs and sternum occurring around the seventh or eighth week of embryonic life.

Lungs

Motility movement and test

The lung's normal motility movement is a downward movement followed by an external rotation.

To evaluate the lungs' motility, the osteopath places his hands on the upper part of each of the patient's hemithoraxes and tests the lungs' motility capacity. He makes sure to be properly rooted inside the pulmonary parenchyma's thickness, starting the evaluation again a few times at different depths if necessary.

It is possible to test the relative motility of the pulmonary lobes, or the possibility of them allowing a sliding movement at the fissures, from the same position (Fig. 6.7).

Motility dysfunction

A lung, under a motility loss, is in an extension dysfunction state and is restricted in its downward movement and external rotation movement.

Normalization

Normalizing the lung's motility is usually carried out in the natural direction, but the normalization should be adapted according to the dysfunction's characteristics. For example, the dysfunction could be an energy-deficiency dysfunction.

Links with traditional Chinese medicine

When linked to an emotion, dysfunctions of the lungs can be associated with sadness, as are those of the colon.

Pleurae

Motility movement and test

The osteopath evaluates the two pleurae one after the other. He must find the specific depth for their distinct evaluation. The inflation factor of the

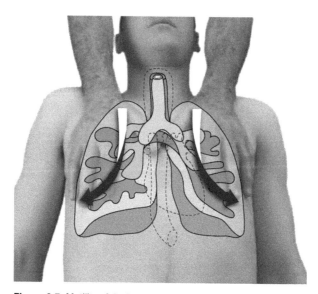

Figure 6.7. Motility of the lungs.

flexion movement helps to determine which pleura he will act on.

The parietal pleura follows the movement of the lateral folds which closes the thorax laterally. Thus, the costal parietal pleura's normal motility movement is a rotation, first outward, then frontward, and finally going toward the anterior line to its folding point. It then becomes the mediastinal parietal pleura to the hilum. The anterior limits of the parietal pleurae are located on each side of the sternum. On the anterior face of the thorax, the right pleura never touches the left pleura. On the posterior face, though, the interpleural ligament connects them, passing in front of the aorta but behind the esophagus at the level of the eighth dorsal vertebra.

The visceral pleura follows the pulmonary parenchyma's development. Its normal motility movement is an outward rotation movement (opposite of the parietal pleura's) and a downward movement.

To evaluate the motility of the pleurae, the osteopath places his hands on the lateral part of each of the patient's hemithoraxes and tests the pleurae's motility capacity.

An easier way to evaluate the entire surface of the pleurae is to perform the test with the subject in a sitting position. The osteopath can then evaluate the parietal pleura from its most posterior part by placing one hand at the level of D8 (interpleural ligament) and another on the sternum where it connects with the anterior pleural recess.

In this test (Fig. 6.8):
- During flexion, the costal parietal pleura moves laterally in its posterior part and rolls up frontward. To gather all the information on the

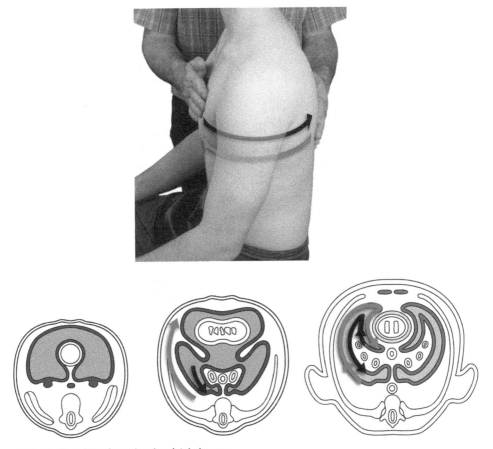

Figure 6.8. Motility of the visceral and parietal pleurae.

pleura's motility, its movement toward the hilum must then be specifically evaluated;

• The osteopath then reaches slightly deeper to evaluate the entire surface of the visceral pleura. During flexion, parameters are inverted in relation to the parietal pleura: the visceral pleura moves laterally in its anterior part and rolls up backward.

Because they are closely linked, the visceral pleura's motility is usually evaluated at the same time as the motility of the lungs.

Motility dysfunction

Pleurae, under a motility loss, are in an extension dysfunction state and are restricted in their respective rotation movements.

Normalization

Normalizing the motility of the pleurae is usually carried out in the natural direction (induction).

Osteopathic considerations

Dysfunctions of the pleurae are common. A hindered differential movement between the two, or between the parietal pleura and the rib cage, can be found during evaluation even if the subject is not aware of any pulmonary pathology. For example, episodes of coughing, with or without fever, that might have seemed insignificant could be the source of osteopathic dysfunctions. Each structure should be tested separately: parenchyma, visceral pleura, parietal pleura, and ribs.

Links with the consequences of pulmonary pathologies

Pleurisy, which causes an abnormal volume of fluid to accumulate in the pleural cavity, can cause a blockage of one pleura in relation to the other. The 'primary' pleura can be either one of the pleurae and its dysfunction might resist a conventional osteopathic treatment that does not sufficiently distinguish between both pleurae.

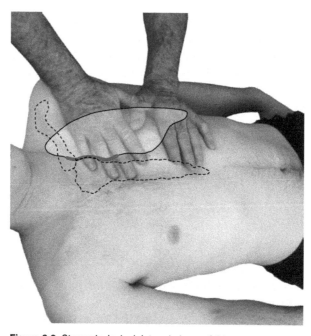

Figure 6.9. Sternoclavicular joint and pleurae fold.

Bronchiolitis and pneumonia affect and frequently hinder the motility of the pulmonary parenchyma. They can have multiple effects, as described by classical osteopathy: tensions of the pleural dome, costal dysfunctions, restrictions in the pleural recesses, etc. It is very important to check for the long-term effects of restrictions on the pulmonary parenchyma established in childhood, especially during growth spurts.

Links with the upper limb

The point where the parietal pleura becomes the mediastinal pleura is located behind the sternoclavicular joint. Chronic motility dysfunctions affecting this region can sometimes have mechanical consequences on the joint and possibly on the entire mechanism of the shoulder complex. They can also have hemodynamic consequences on the upper limb, which are precursors to arthrosis, especially around the thumb and wrist (rhizarthrosis) (Fig. 6.9).

The lung as a pressure column

When the all of the pulmonary parenchyma and all of the pleurae on one side are restricted in their motility, the hemithorax sometimes acts like a rigid pressure column. Often, in such cases, the hemithorax will have suffered high-speed trauma, such as a car accident while wearing a seatbelt, which has made the lung twist around its vertical axis. In such cases, the pleural dome, the lung's upper insertion, must be examined for classic symptoms, such as cervicodorsal pain, cervicobrachialgia and effects on the stellate ganglion. The lower part of the lung, where the liver, stomach, and kidneys – under the usual negative pressure of the thorax and thus significantly affected by restrictions of the hemithorax – are hindered in their normal physiology, must also be examined. Understanding this particular situation is essential for creating a proper treatment plan to restore the motility and mobility of the thorax.

Chapter 7

Digestive System

Summary

This chapter focuses initially on embryological generalities relating to the digestive system before going on
to give an outline of its neurological organization in
order to explain the links between the visceral sphere
and the central nervous system and musculoskeletal system. The digestive system is one of the most
common reasons for consultation in clinical practice,
greatly exceeding consultations for localized reasons;
improving its functioning is essential to many aspects
of health.

The organs and viscera are presented in order according to the direction of transit. For each of the organs
and viscera, tests and normalization techniques are presented, along with osteopathic considerations on the
consequences of their motility dysfunctions.

The digestive system is of the utmost importance
for the organism's health. It is often subject to
dysfunctions directly affecting its physiology and
causing local signs and symptoms, but visceral
dysfunctions can also have remote consequences
affecting the musculoskeletal system via tissular
links (for example, ligament attachments), or via
nervous links (for example, viscerosomatic reflexes
or referred cutaneous pain). The analysis framework used inembryological motility work adds a
whole new level of work for these more traditional
considerations and introduces newer and closer
links between the visceral sphere and the central
nervous system.

The visceral sphere also entertains close links
with nutrition as well as elements of traditional
Chinese medicine. To document these links
between Chinese medicine and osteopathy, classical correlations between organs and viscera and
emotions are used. These correlations must be
considered with tact and respect in the clinical
context because emotional states are not easy to
interpret, especially when emotions have been
somatized and remain unconscious. Obviously,
Chinese medicine is much more complex and subtle than these few connections suggest, but being
familiar with them is clinically useful and provides
a foundation for the acquisition of further
knowledge.

For each of the organs or viscera, elements of
classical anatomy and physiology will be briefly
outlined for each of the organs and viscera.
Further information can be found in classical
medical and osteopathic sources, and an exhaustive
knowledge of anatomy, physiology, and physiopa-
thology is the only way to make sure all the necessary clinical connections are accounted for.

Embryological generalities

The thoracic, caudal and lateral plications of the
embryo transform the trilaminar disc into a complex structure consisting of three tubes that fit
inside one another, with the internal one (the
endoderm) eventually forming the primitive
digestive tract.

In the development of the abdomen, the container is established before its contents. During
the lateral plications, the parietal peritoneum
and the walls of the abdomen are established
before the viscera and the definitive visceral peritoneum. The only exception to this principle is
the very last midline closure at the umbilicus.

At first, the digestive tract is rectilinear and
linked to the posterior wall of the embryo by the
long dorsal mesentery. Also related to the posterior

wall is the primitive aorta, source of the arterial branches associated with each part of the primitive intestine, the foregut, the midgut, and the hindgut.

The foregut starts at the oropharyngeal membrane (which will become the buccal cavity) and ends at the major duodenal papilla or ampulla of Vater (which will become the terminal part of the duct of Wirsung and the common bile duct). The foregut includes the thoracic and abdominal parts of the esophagus, the stomach, the upper half of the duodenum, the exocrine and endocrine pancreas, and the gall bladder.

The midgut follows on from the foregut. Opened on the yolk sac at the beginning of its development, the midgut will provide the lower half of the duodenum, the small intestine, the cecum, the ascending colon, and approximately two-thirds of the transverse colon to the definitive digestive system.

The hindgut ends at the cloacal membrane (which will become the anus). It will become the last third of the transverse colon, the descending and sigmoid colons, and the rectum.

The three-branched celiac trunk provides blood irrigation to the inferior part of the foregut and the superior part of the midgut. The superior mesenteric artery irrigates the remaining midgut and the inferior mesenteric artery irrigates the hindgut.

The demarcation between the midgut and hindgut is also the boundary between the two sources of parasympathetic innervation in the digestive tract (cranial and sacral sources).

Originally rectilinear, the digestive tract will become more and more complex as the organs and viscera develop and reach their definitive form and situation. Not only is this growth establishing all the elements of the digestive tract, but it is also the origin of what will be the arrangement of the parts of the visceral peritoneum that will form the mesenteries, omenta, fasciae, and ligaments. The parts of the peritoneum and their arrangement are also important for understanding the mobility of organs and viscera and also the vascularization of the elements of the digestive tract, for which they provide support.

Neurological regulation of the intestinal tract

Describing each of the elements of the visceral sphere is only useful if its nervous regulation system is properly understood, since neurological information is essential to the digestive system's regular functions. Links between the intestinal tract and the brain have been frequently researched in recent scientific literature, under the term 'brain–gut axis' or visceral brain (Bonaz 2010). These communications between the central nervous system and the gastro-intestinal tract have to be integrated into clinical reasoning processes in order to properly link signs and symptoms to the osteopathic dysfunctions found during evaluation.

Most of the regulation of visceral functioning happens locally. The enteric nervous system regulates the visceral functions with independent actions. It is made up of 100 million sensory neurons located inside the walls of the organs, arranged as Meissner's plexus (submucous plexus) and Auerbach's plexus (myenteric plexus). These plexuses form a reticular tissue resembling that of the brain, explaining their 'visceral brain' title. This system manages local reflexes and visceral activity coordination, but it is not directly concerned with pain-related information, except when the secretory activity is affected (Yamada et al. 2003).

The functioning of the digestive system is completed by local hormonal control (Marieb 2005). Hormones, often resembling those of the central nervous system, are directly secreted by the digestive tract's walls, considered the biggest endocrine organ in the body (Yamada et al. 2003). The proper functioning of the digestive system is also ensured by an adequate gut flora (Matricon et al. 2010) and by activation of lymphocytes by the immune system in the presence of antigens.

Only a small proportion of information needs to be transmitted to the central nervous system for it to coordinate its neurovegetative actions according to the needs of the different parts of the digestive tract and the needs of other parts of the body. In normal conditions, the brain is permanently but unconsciously kept informed of the functioning of the digestive system. It manages this information with the help of a network involving the hypothalamus, the limbic system, and the cortex (insular, prefrontal, cingulate) to ensure homeostasis (Bonaz 2010).

Sensory visceral information ascending to the central nervous system uses two routes: the vagal pathway and the splanchnic pathway, with both playing complementary but different roles. Nociceptive or inflammatory information is usually transmitted via the splanchnic pathway, which is also related to effects of stress, while physiological information, such as distension or information pertaining to ingested nutrients, is transmitted via the vagal pathway. These two neurological transmission pathways can be either facilitated or inhibited and are often under the influence of the emotional state and the effects of behavior (Grundy 2002).

In pathological conditions, visceral information can become conscious, especially in inflammatory conditions or in certain chronic pain conditions.

Chronic pain of the digestive system can be caused by intense inflammatory phenomena or by significant and often surgery-related traumas. In some cases, hyperalgesia or painful sensations are involved, even when the stimulus that caused them was painless. These types of pain are hard to medically investigate because they are vague and are often linked to particular psychological states (Matricon et al. 2010).

In these cases of chronic pain, medullar neurological pathways are sensitive and overactive. They contribute to the amplification of the pain signal at the central level. This signal can be referred to both the digestive system and the somatic level (for example, cutaneous modifications) (Verne et al. 2001), paving the way for chronification.

Chronic pain can also be explained by a decrease in the superior centers' inhibition capacity for visceral pain (information coming from the brainstem and the brain). This inhibition deficit can be caused by hypervigilance following a recurring painful disorder, by a significant pathological stress incurred in childhood, such as sexual abuse, or by intense and recent stress sources preceding the chronic visceral pain (Matricon et al. 2010).

Beside effects on the central nervous system (see the section on the first fold in Chapter 5), four zones must be investigated in relation to neurological regulation of the visceral sphere: the segmental vertebral/costal level, the jugular foramen, the sacrum, and the walls of the organs and viscera.

Segmental vertebral/ costal level

A viscerosomatic reflex can be initiated by visceral information travelling in the afferent fibers (50% of the splanchnic nervous pathway) (Bonaz 2010). This reflex can cause a 'neurological lens' phenomenon in the corresponding metamere, inducing dermatome, sclerotome, or myotome disorders (Korr 1996). These paravertebral muscular tensions can cause vertebral somatic or isolated costal dysfunctions – a preferential vertebral dysfunction – or dysfunctions affecting a group of vertebrae related to the same nervous plexus.

A vertebral or costal group can, in the other direction, cause a dysfunction in the autonomous nervous system and, eventually, a visceral dysfunction. From experience, it seems that the neurological organization of the plexus is often successful in offsetting the effects of a segmental somatic dysfunction, and so the resulting visceral disorders do not systematically appear.

Links with the cranial base and the jugular foramen

Influxes from the upper part of the digestive tract (up to the transverse colon) can pass up to the jugular foramen through the vagus nerve, where they relay through the nervous ganglia functionally reacting to the intensity of the information; 90% of the information in the vagus nerve is afferent and sensory (Bonaz 2010). In clinical practice, it has often been observed that an excessively intense influx can cause an overload in the nervous ganglia of the jugular foramen, which can over time cause the emergence of a dysfunction of the jugular foramen, thus restraining the freedom of the cranial base on the same side. Finding the affected side is possible via palpation only, the two vagus nerves sharing information along their exocranial paths; under the bronchi and up to the target organs, the two vagus nerves are so interconnected that they can even be considered as a plexus (Guibert and Guibert 1973).

Conversely, a dysfunction of the jugular foramen can affect the vagus nerve and negatively impact the visceral functions.

Links with the sacrum

Influxes from the lower part of the digestive tract (transverse colon, descending colon, sigmoid, and rectum) are linked to the sacral S2 to S4 levels. A caudal plication in an extension dysfunction state can sometimes impair the functioning of these organs.

Walls of the viscera and organs

With the enteric nervous system being located in the walls of the viscera and organs, normal motility of the latter is essential for proper neurological regulation of the visceral function.

Esophagus

The esophagus follows a long vertical axis, with slight curves. Its elongated 'S' shape allows for a certain elongation capacity.

To understand the importance of the esophagus, it is essential to consider the muscular and aponeurotic continuity starting from the base of the cranium (the pharynx's constrictor muscles), then moving into the esophagus itself following the cervicodorsal part of the vertebral column to D3, and finally passing through the phrenic center with a privileged link with the left crus firmly inserted to the left on L2 (partly freeing L3).

Linking many structures, this tissular continuity explains many functional disorders involving mechanical and tissular dysfunctions or viscerosomatic/somatovisceral relations between the various elements.

The esophagus' function is to ensure food passage from the mouth to the stomach. The junction between those two viscera is the cardia, at the opening of the stomach, but the lower sphincter of the esophagus is what actually ensures continence.

The basic tonus of the lower sphincter of the esophagus is ensured by the effect of the orthosympathetic system coming from the vertebral D5–D6 level. This nervous effect is potentiated by the action of gastrin. The action of the lower sphincter of the esophagus is mechanically induced by the diaphragm's contraction during inspiration and the ascent of the fundus of the stomach that closes the angle of His during diaphragmatic expiration, if this angle is respected.

While the diaphragm moves, the sphincter of the esophagus stays still and the diaphragm slides around it, physiologically restricted in its amplitude by the phrenoesophageal ligaments. The area in which the esophagus goes through the diaphragm is prone to restrictions and motility blockages of both structures. A lack of coherence in the physiology of both structures can cause hiatal hernias (with or without reflux) and complications altering the structure of the mucous membrane of the esophagus. Such dysfunctions usually cause significant pain. However, the diagnostic impression should not be based on painful phenomena alone, because sometimes dysfunctions exist without prompting local pain. Such alterations in the mucous membrane can be a precursor of cancer, which can appear even without pain or discomfort (Nason et al. 2011). In these situations, the identification of a functional disorder by the osteopath can be an important preventive tool.

Embryological movement

The esophagus develops from the foregut and is established in the same direction as the thoracic plication (a cephalocaudal movement).

Motility movement and test

The flexion motility movement of the esophagus is a downward movement.

For the upper part of the esophagus, the downward movement is tested by a direct contact at the left anterior C6 level.

For the lower part of the esophagus, the downward movement is tested in the projection of the esophagus passing through the diaphragm, at the left K6 junction with the sternum. The osteopath places both hands, leaving between them an esophagus-wide space. The motility is specifically tested for each side of the esophagus. A restriction in one of the sides can lead to a rolling hernia, and a restriction in both sides is most likely to lead to a sliding hernia.

The osteopath tests for the presence of the complete motility movement of the esophagus (Fig. 7.1).

Motility dysfunction

The esophagus, under a motility loss, is in an extension dysfunction state and is restricted in its downward movement.

Normalization

Normalizing the esophagus is usually carried out in the natural direction (induction).

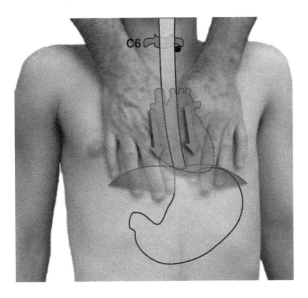

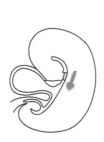

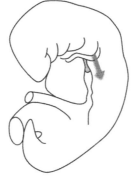

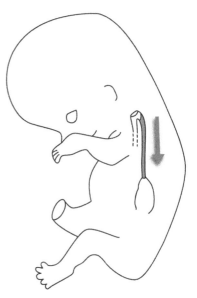

Figure 7.1. Motility of the esophagus.

Links with traditional Chinese medicine

When associated with an emotion, dysfunctions of the esophagus and stomach are linked to anxiety.

Osteopathic considerations

Often underestimated, the esophagus is an extremely important structure, with its testing and normalization being useful for a variety of reasons in consultations. Treating the esophagus can often provide original solutions for vertebral column problems, digestive function disorders or cranial mechanism disorders. Given its situation and depth, the results achieved through embryological motility work are far superior to those achieved using classical techniques.

Links with the vertebral column

The esophagus is closely linked to the cervicodorsal column; it can bring it forward or into compression when dysfunctional, thus causing multiple adaptation dysfunctions and their numerous vertebral symptoms. Although not constant, this dysfunctional schema can spread via tissular continuity with the diaphragm and the left crus until it causes an extension of L2, which is subjected to the greater part of the mechanical traction of the crus.

Links with digestive function

An extension motility dysfunction of the esophagus is an essential element of the symptomatic hiatal hernia. Only treating dysfunctions of the stomach and nervous afferences is not sufficient to put a definitive end to signs and symptoms.

Refluxes indicate more complex dysfunctional schemas, simultaneously involving tissular, mechanical, hormonal, and nervous factors.

The area of the lower esophageal sphincter is closely linked to the apex of the heart. In the case of, for example, refluxes or significant digestive discomfort, this should be taken into account when faced with chronic signs and symptoms pertaining to the lower esophageal sphincter. These types of dysfunctions seem to be related to a very significant restriction in the heart's torsion movement (and are thus also related to the establishment of the apex).

Links with the cranial base

Dysfunctions of the upper attachments of the esophagus can cause, via tissular continuity, blockages of the cranial base that are more frequently or intensely located to the left. With the chronicity factor, these tensions can spread their dysfunctional influence to all of the cranial base and impair the flexion mechanism, leading to consequences that are well-known in classical cranial osteopathy.

In clinical practice, it has been possible to attribute some cases of left-sided facial paralysis to a seemingly primary motility dysfunction of the esophagus. Disorders located at the left of the cranial base, involving the temporal and occipital bones, have been resolved by working on the esophagus. The presumed effect can be explained by the link between the posterior belly of the digastric muscle and the facial nerve opening in the stylohyoid foramen.

Stomach

The stomach is a bulge of the digestive system that serves as a temporary container for food and fluids, mixing, kneading, and stirring them. It also absorbs vitamin B12. The stomach secretes hormones that regulate the transit of food, often the same hormones as used by the central nervous system. Gastrin stimulates acid production in the stomach's walls, responding to distension. It increases the intestinal motricity and blood flow of the digestive tract.

Embryological movement

The stomach develops from the foregut. Two complementary movements occur during its embryological development.

The first movement is a rotation that moves the posterior part of the stomach from the center to the left along an axis that passes through both ends: the cardia and the pylorus. Elongation of the posterior mesogastrium is essential to this movement.

The second movement in the establishment of the stomach is around an anteroposterior axis represented by the celiac trunk. The stomach bud rotates clockwise while increasing in volume. The dorsal curve grows more and becomes the greater curve, while the ventral curve becomes the lesser curve.

The combination of these two movements gives the stomach its definitive shape and position.

Motility movement and test

The stomach's flexion motility movement is a rotation from left to right along an axis that passes through both ends, and another rotation along the anteroposterior axis (celiac trunk). The complete motility movement is the result of both movements.

To evaluate the stomach's motility, the osteopath locates the transverse colon to position himself in the supramesocolic cavity, of which all of the left part is occupied by the stomach.

The osteopath places his hands on the rib cage and feels the stomach's complete motility movement (Fig. 7.2).

To specifically test the mesogastrium, the patient is placed in a sitting position. The osteopath places one hand on the medial dorsal region and another on the anterolateral part of the rib cage to feel the elongation of the mesogastrium's complete motility movement.

Motility dysfunction

The stomach, under a motility loss, is in an extension dysfunction state and is restricted in the amplitude of one or both of its embryological establishing movements.

Normalization

Normalizing the stomach's motility is usually carried out in the natural direction (induction), but the normalization is selected according to the characteristics of the dysfunction. For example, the dysfunction could be an energy-deficiency dysfunction, although these are clinically uncommon.

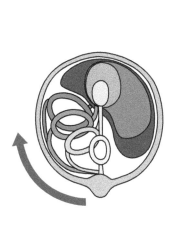
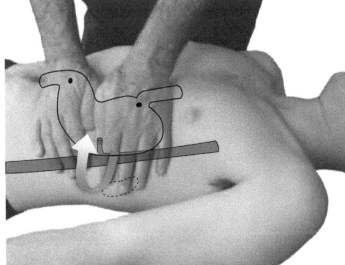

Figure 7.2. Motility of the stomach.

If the motility restriction is not too significant, work on both of the stomach's movements will usually be sufficient for proper normalization. If restoring a perfect movement is problematic, verifying the mesogastrium may often prove useful; indeed, it has to be able to elongate and move from the center to the left to allow for the stomach's proper motility. Significant restrictions of the mesogastrium can be secondary to a motility dysfunction of the spleen, which develops from the mesoderm.

Links with traditional Chinese medicine

When associated with an emotion, dysfunctions of the esophagus and stomach are linked to anxiety.

Osteopathic considerations

Links with the digestive function

Extension dysfunctions of the stomach can cause an increase in the intensity of digestive discomfort linked to an extension dysfunction of the esophagus, as described in the last section.

Motility dysfunctions of the stomach can cause dyspepsia and gastritis, possibly resulting in ulceration when sufficiently intense.

Links with the musculoskeletal system

Dysfunctions of the stomach can also be the starting point for many disorders of the musculoskeletal system. By reflex, they can cause left paravertebral dorsalgia between D5 and D9. They can also be related to a lumbar pain to the left, often located at L1–L2. These pains are related to blockages in the cupola and left crus of the diaphragm, thus directly pertaining to the stomach's physiology. When the pylorus is dysfunctional, it causes right lumbar pain with a dysfunction precisely located to the right at L1. This dysfunction often appears in people who are in the habit of eating too fast. When faced with a dysfunction of the stomach, all the motor and sensory signs and symptoms pertaining to L1 and L2 must be closely examined.

Middle back pain usually located to the left can be linked to severe restrictions of the posterior mesogastrium's motility.

Links with anxiety and stress response

Even if precise tissular osteopathic mobility work of the stomach often achieves worthwhile results, the embryological motility approach for this organ is especially useful because it seems that contemporary lifestyles in the Western world make its inhabitants particularly prone to frequent and often improperly managed anxiety disorders. Anxiety is the source of numerous motility dysfunctions of the stomach and the esophagus that are hard to relieve without a therapeutic means of directly treating the source of the anxiety. It is then essential, when establishing a proper intervention plan, to understand the organism's stress response and to add central nervous system work to visceral work. It is also of the utmost importance to take the patient's lifestyle into account and to evaluate, according to tissular responses, the current state of the anxiety disorder; whether the anxiety disorder is active or resolved will greatly affect the therapeutic approach and the sustainability of the improvements.

Liver

The importance of the largest gland in the human body, involved in almost 700 roles and functions, is well established in medicine. For further information, the reader should refer to classical physiology textbooks. Clinically, it is essential to keep in mind the significant role of the liver in the general circulation and the assimilation of nutrients, as well as its emunctory function. Specifically, the right lobe of the liver ensures the 'dietary' function, while the left lobe of the liver focuses more on the excretory function. The left lobe is therefore more subject to the consequences of medication intake or to 'chemical' events in the body: chemotherapy, contact with toxins, exposure to pollution or polluting agents, etc.

Embryological movement

The hepatic bud, at the beginning of its development, appears between the phrenic center and its parietal peritoneum. It develops frontward and downward, modifying the curve of the septum to an inferior concavity. When the hepatic cells meet the anterior wall, they continue to grow toward the right, following the anterolateral wall and occupying the right infradiaphragmatic space. Cellular proliferation transforms the infradiaphragmatic parietal peritoneum into a visceral peritoneum, which envelops the whole surface of the liver apart from a region called the area nuda of which the perimeter forms the coronary ligament.

The liver's movement starts from a posteromedial position. The first movement is posteroanterior, until it joins the abdomen's posterior wall, and the liver then rotates to the right until it joins the right lateral wall and the posterior wall, in that order. The liver's rapid growth allows for blood circulation toward the heart, which can then take care of the needs generated by the brain's equally rapid growth.

Since it develops in the extension of the anterior mesentery linking the stomach to the anterior wall, the liver's growth and rightward displacement initiates the stomach's first movement.

The part of the anterior mesentery located between the stomach and the liver will become the lesser omentum. Due to the rotations of the stomach and the liver, the definitive version of the lesser omentum will hang down from the stomach. These rotations will also cause the formation of the lesser sac. The part of the anterior mesentery located between the liver and the abdomen's anterior wall will become the falciform ligament.

Motility movement and test

The first part of the liver's flexion motility movement is a frontward movement, and the second part is a rotation of a great amplitude to the right.

Evaluating the first motility movement of the liver can be done with the subject in a sitting position or in the dorsal decubitus position. The osteopath places one hand on the dorsal column and another at the epigastrium and/or on the rib cage at the level of the liver. He evaluates the liver's complete movement: first the anteroposterior component, and then the clockwise lateral rotation component. He must evaluate the liver's motility in its entire volume because, for example, the upper part can be under more restrictions than the lower part, or vice versa. He must also consider the specific movements of the right and left lobes (Fig. 7.3).

Motility dysfunction

The liver, under a motility loss, is in an extension dysfunction state and is restricted in one or many of the components of its normal movement.

Normalization

Normalizing the liver's motility is usually carried out in the natural direction (induction), but the normalization is selected according to the characteristics of the dysfunction. An energy-efficiency dysfunction is an example of the type of dysfunction that might occur, although this is clinically uncommon. In such cases, it is necessary to check for pre-existing medical conditions that might be the source of the dysfunction.

Links with traditional Chinese medicine

When associated with an emotion, dysfunctions of the liver are linked to anger. They can also be linked to serious emotional troubles because the liver is an essential element in general emotional equilibrium, and absorbs the 'excess.' It is said, in Chinese medicine, that the liver can take energy from the brain. Treating the liver is therefore essential in cases of mental fatigue and depression.

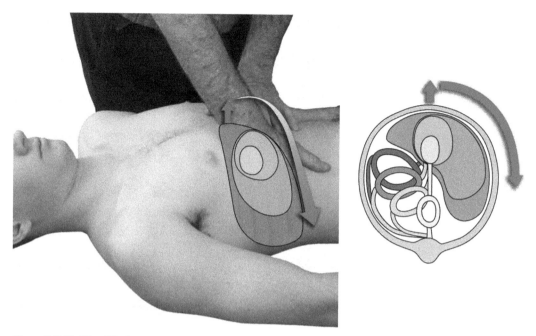

Figure 7.3. Motility of the liver.

Osteopathic considerations

The high frequency of hepatic dysfunctions justifies exhaustive research on anatomy, physiology and the links to clinical signs, which are often significant and sometimes severe. The importance of the liver in health makes its therapeutic approach fundamental to osteopathy. Direct and distant links between the liver and the rest of the body are so numerous that synthesizing them succinctly is difficult. Osteopathic tissular techniques for the mobility dysfunctions of the liver are often effective in improving the quantitative metrics of the thoracic breathing movements or in normalizing the links with the adjacent viscera, but they often lack the capacity to restore the vitality of the tissues. It is therefore difficult to normalize the liver's functions in the long term, as well as to 're-energize' the liver, without the contribution of visceral motility techniques.

There is a big difference between the liver's mobility and its motility movement – which is not the case for many organs or viscera – and this could be one of the reasons that explains the great disparity in the results of embryology-based motility techniques. These differences are found especially when working on vascular functions and the general state. Once the liver's motility is restored, classical osteopathic techniques for the tissular environment can treat hepatic mobility dysfunctions in an easier way.

Vascular importance

A significant blood influx of 2,000 liters passes through the liver in 24 hours; 70 per cent of this influx comes from the hepatic portal system and the remaining 30 per cent, from the hepatic artery. A proper energetic function of the hepatic parenchyma eases the intrahepatic blood circulation. The liver's normalization is therefore essential for all attempts at general circulation recovery, and it must, in most cases, be completed by normalization of the entire diaphragmatic function.

As classically described in osteopathy, the vascular influence of the liver is felt, via the arrangement of the mesenteries, up to the left iliac fossa. When the liver is obstructed, circulatory signs are often found; these are characterized by a secondary congestion of the iliac vessels, and therefore by frequent hemorrhoids, constipation, and the formation of varicose veins in the left lower limb. The iliac bone is under 'vascular pressure' and its normalization might be difficult in this situation.

Because the inferior vena cava runs along the entire posterosuperior face of the liver, the latter can disrupt circulation inside the inferior vena cava as soon as it is congested; signs and symptoms will then be bilateral. As a direct consequence, this disruption will cause the feeling of heavy legs, congestion in the lesser pelvis and, if sufficiently intense, congestion in the organs for which return circulation depends on the liver. Hepatic congestion, when associated with portal system congestion, can cause a secondary congestion in the small intestine that should be considered when evaluating. The global pressure in the abdomen will then be modified.

Blockages of the cervicodorsal junction and the first two ribs can be linked to a vascular deficiency of the liver, causing an overload in the azygos venous system in charge of draining this region. An overloaded azygos system can be responsible for improper drainage of the head. These symptoms, when present, provide a hint to the practitioner of the presence of a vascular hepatic dysfunction.

Links with the musculoskeletal system

As the diaphragmatic parietal peritoneum related to the liver is innervated by the phrenic nerve, the effects of a liver dysfunction can be felt in the shoulder and neck region where the liver creates referred pain via the metameric link.

Certain hepatic tissular modifications, sometimes secondary to chronic motility dysfunctions, cause a reaction in the right diaphragmatic cupola along with a secondary tension surge in the right crus of the diaphragm, causing mechanical dysfunctions at L3 on the right (the last vertebra to which the right crus extends). L3 being responsible for the deep sensitivity of the knee, the liver is therefore often the primary cause of pain in the right knee for which the clinically observed mechanical components cannot explain the extent and persistence of the signs and symptoms.

Effects on the emunctories

The accumulation of toxins of a dietary, environmental or medicinal origin in the liver can trigger side effects on the skin when they are released in the blood. This effect is sometimes noticeable after osteopathic treatment. The liver can therefore play a role in some types of asthma and eczema. In these cases, the best solution is sometimes provided by work on the gall bladder, which helps hepatic detoxification.

Duodenum

Classically, the duodenum is divided into four parts, but this more of an anatomical than a physiological reality. Physiologically, the duodenum is composed rather of two distinct parts, divided by the ampulla of Vater. The superior part (first part and proximal part of the second part) is functionally linked to the stomach, and is part of the foregut from an embryological viewpoint. The inferior part (distal part of the second, third and fourth parts) is linked to the small intestine, and is part of the midgut from an embryological viewpoint.

The duodenum secretes multiple hormones (serotonin, dopamine, gastrin, motilin, etc.) and digestive enzymes; 75 to 80 per cent of absorbed calcium is absorbed by the inferior part of the duodenum.

Embryological movement

The duodenum develops simultaneously from the foregut and the midgut. The medial line and equilibrium point between the two is the ampulla of Vater.

As they develop from two distinct embryological structures, both parts also perform distinct movements. The superior part of the duodenum follows the stomach and the inferior part follows the small intestine.

The foregut, from the duodenum to the ampulla of Vater, rotates clockwise around a sagittal axis represented by the celiac trunk.

The midgut, from the ampulla of Vater to the small intestine, rotates counterclockwise around a sagittal axis represented by the superior mesenteric artery.

The combination of these movements causes the typical 'C' shape of the duodenum.

Motility movement and test

The flexion motility movement of the superior part of the duodenum is a clockwise rotation.

The flexion motility movement of the inferior part of the duodenum is a counterclockwise rotation.

The general 'C' shape of the duodenum therefore seems to close during the flexion motility movement.

The ampulla of Vater, a point of equilibrium between the superior and inferior parts, does not move on the high/low axis but will move from the anterior part of the duodenum to the posterior part following the lower bile duct and the exocrine pancreatic duct. It is found at the internal face of the duodenum in its definitive version, when it has achieved its final 'C' shape.

To evaluate to duodenum's motility, the osteopath stands to the left of the patient and finds the ampulla of Vater. He places one hand on top of it and the other below, with the index fingers framing the ampulla of Vater. If standing to the right of the patient, the osteopath frames the ampulla of Vater using both thumbs. He evaluates the duodenum's motility capacity. Both parts of the duodenum must be equally motile and their movements must be synced (Fig. 7.4).

Motility dysfunction

The duodenum, under a motility loss, is in an extension dysfunction state and is restricted in the movement of its superior part, its inferior part, or in both parts.

Normalization

Normalizing the duodenum is usually carried out in the natural direction (induction).

Links with traditional Chinese medicine

When associated with an emotion, dysfunctions of the superior part of the duodenum, as with the

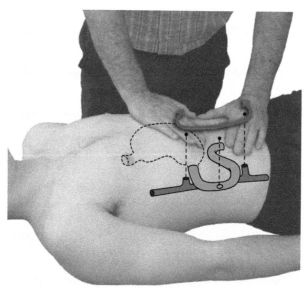

Figure 7.4. Motility of the duodenum

esophagus and stomach, are linked to anxiety. Dysfunctions of the inferior part, as with the small intestine, are instead linked to joy or the absence of joy.

Osteopathic considerations

Given its position and physiology, the duodenum's motility restrictions are often secondary to its environment, and an isolated dysfunction is uncommon. For example, the first part of the duodenum is often restricted by dysfunctions of the stomach. The therapeutic approach for the duodenum will therefore often consider the esophagus–stomach–duodenum continuum, the liver–gallbladder pair, the duodenum's close relationship with the pancreas or its relationship with the mesenteric root and the ligament of Treitz.

However, a hyperstimulation of the ganglion impar, located in front of the coccyx, can cause a pelvic and abdominal vasoconstriction, with most extensive consequences affecting the duodenum, given its significant vascularization. In this situation, the duodenum feels very rigid under palpation.

Gallbladder, upper and lower bile ducts, and exocrine pancreas

Essential functions of the gallbladder include emulsion of fats and detoxification of the liver. Bile also allows for the regularization of the bowel transit, the elimination of bilirubin, and the absorption of fat-soluble vitamins.

The exocrine part of the pancreas, linked to the ventral pancreatic bud, ensures digestive functions by the secretion of pancreatic juices.

Embryological movement

The gallbladder and the pancreas both come from the foregut.

The cystic diverticulum is linked to the ampulla of Vater by the bile duct, where the ventral pancreatic bud is also found.

The ventral pancreatic bud, initially located on the ventral face of the duodenum, rotates by 180 degrees to migrate toward the dorsal pancreatic bud, which is related to the endocrine function. Combined, they form the head of the pancreas. The lower bile duct and exocrine pancreatic duct's embryological movement is then completed, even if two additional factors need to be considered in order to understand their final arrangement. As a matter of fact, these structures follow the duodenum's displacement (the 'C' shaped curve that sets the vertical part of the duodenum to the right of the medial line and the complete duodenum closer to the posterior wall in the definitive body). They will also follow the displacement of the dorsal pancreatic bud.

During its development, the gallbladder ascends toward the liver, reaching its position at the inferior face. Over the course of this movement, the bile duct is elongated in two different directions: the upper bile duct (or hepatic duct) follows the ascending movement of the gallbladder, while the lower bile duct follows the ventral pancreatic bud's migration, reaching the internal face of the duodenum.

Motility movement and test

The flexion motility movement of the ventral pancreatic bud, precursor of the **exocrine function of the pancreas**, is a 180-degree rotation around a vertical axis represented by the duodenum, going from the latter's anterior face to its posterior face. This rotation movement occurs around the ampulla of Vater, which represents its fixed point. The exocrine pancreas then follows the 'C' shaped curvature movement of the duodenum, in which the originally anterior face of the duodenum becomes its external face, and the originally posterior face becomes its internal face, in the definitive version. Taking these positions into account, testing the motility movement of the exocrine pancreas around the duodenum is carried out by evaluating the movement that goes from the external face of the duodenum to its internal face, passing underneath it.

The **lower bile duct** is tested at the same time as the exocrine duct of the pancreas. It follows, in its flexion motility movement, the ventral pancreatic bud; in doing so, it elongates.

To evaluate the motility of the exocrine pancreatic duct and lower bile duct, the osteopath places one hand on the second part of the duodenum and tests the capacity of the lower bile duct and exocrine duct to move from the external to the internal face of the duodenum, by passing underneath it.

The **gallbladder's** flexion motility movement is an upward movement under the liver, causing the elongation of the **upper bile duct** (or hepatic duct).

To evaluate the motility of the gallbladder and upper bile duct, the osteopath places one hand on the liver and another on the second part of the duodenum. He tests the gallbladder's motility capacity and its synchronism with the rotation of the liver.

The synchronism between the movements of the gallbladder and pancreatic duct and that of the duodenum is sometimes worth investigating, but checking the synchronism between the gallbladder's movement and the liver's movement is even more important, because this is the most frequent source of dysfunctions. It is generally necessary to check this region as a whole to ensure each structure's optimal function (Fig. 7.5).

Motility dysfunction

The lower bile duct and the exocrine pancreas, under a motility loss, are in an extension dysfunction state and their rotation movement around the duodenum, when passing underneath it, is incomplete.

The upper bile duct and the gallbladder, under a motility loss, are in an extension dysfunction state and their upward movement is either incomplete or out of sync with the liver's movement.

Normalization

Normalizing the motility of the gallbladder, the bile ducts and the exocrine pancreas is usually carried out in the natural direction, while ensuring their synchronism, especially between the bile ducts/gallbladder and the liver. For these structures, the normalization technique must sometimes be selected according to the characteristics of the dysfunction.

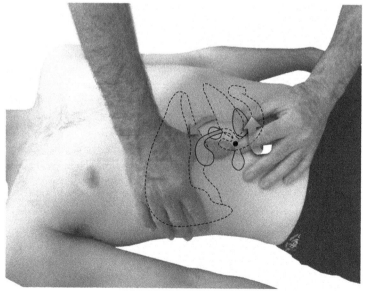
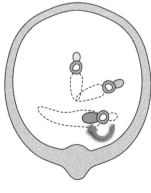

Figure 7.5. Motility of the gallbladder, bile ducts, and exocrine pancreas.

Links with traditional Chinese medicine

When associated with an emotion, dysfunctions of the gallbladder and exocrine pancreas are linked to the decision-making process. It is useful to recall that bile is very significant in Chinese medicine, which considers it as an equivalent to blood.

Osteopathic considerations

Links with the digestive function

Physiology indicates that 20 per cent of toxins are excreted via the blood, while 80 per cent are excreted via the digestive tract – a fact that emphasizes how important it is that the gallbladder functions correctly. A dysfunction of the gallbladder can cause the accumulation of toxins in the blood and in the liver, which are eventually deposited in the soft tissues, especially the muscles and tendons. An accumulation of toxins causes erratic pains varying in intensity, unrelated to any precise mechanical pattern and therefore without any logical link to an activity. It also predisposes to sprains and tendonitis. These signs and symptoms may be linked to Chinese medicine which states that the liver and gallbladder regulate the energy of the muscles and tendons. When toxins are not stored in the muscles and tendons, they can migrate to the skin, where they cause pruritus and cutaneous conditions.

Before regulating the gallbladder or aiming for detoxification of the liver, it is essential to check for correct movement of the bile ducts and that the duodenum is functioning properly to ensure the circulatory freedom of the bile toward the digestive tract. Detoxifying the liver requires caution because a sudden influx of toxins in the blood may lead to the rapid occurrence of pruritis, as described previously. With a carefully planned therapeutic intervention, this inconvenience can be avoided.

In some cases, lithiasis may be caused solely by local dysfunctions of the gallbladder. Lithiasis is very common, but it is asymptomatic in 70–80 per cent of cases. In industrialized countries, gallstones are most often formed by cholesterol derivatives (Yamada et al. 2003). They are related to dietary, hormonal, and genetic risk factors and they are more frequent in multiparous women (Régent et al. 2006). A fascial link might be the cause of this higher rate of occurrence of gallstones in women compared to men. In fact, some gallstones are found to be clinically related to tension in the inframesenteric fascia that links the uterus to the duodenojejunal flexure that follows the posterior wall of the abdomen.

Under a motility dysfunction of the exocrine pancreas, feces may present an abnormal consistency; they are mushy and greasy, and they float on water.

Links with the gallbladder meridian

The gallbladder meridian is one of the longest in the human body. Its cranial part can cause headaches affecting half of the cranium that need to be distinguished from 'real' migraines.

Endocrine pancreas

The endocrine function of the pancreas is responsible for the production of insulin and glucagon; both hormones regulate blood sugar.

A healthy lifestyle is very important for proper functioning of the endocrine pancreas. Reducing the intake of refined sugar and allowing the digestive system a period of rest in between meals is also very important. Excessive alcohol intake may lead to pancreatitis or lysis of the pancreas by inhibiting the sphincter controlling its access; this allows enterokinase to enter the pancreas and destroy it by triggering a digestive process.

Embryological movement

The dorsal pancreatic bud of the foregut becomes the endocrine pancreas. The dorsal bud is the origin of the body, the tail, and part of the head of the pancreas.

The dorsal pancreatic bud initiates its movement from a position in the sagittal plane, bringing with it the lower bile duct and the ventral pancreatic bud. The establishing movement of the endocrine pancreas is a migration, bringing the head and body toward the posterior wall and the tail toward the left lateral wall. This movement can be globally described as a wide quarter-circle movement bringing the tail of pancreas toward the spleen.

Motility movement and test

The flexion motility movement of the endocrine pancreas is a wide quarter-circle movement to the left.

To evaluate the motility of the endocrine pancreas, if the osteopath is to the left of the subject, he places his fingers on the head of the pancreas and his palm toward the tail. If he is to the right of the subject, he places one hand on the pancreas, placing the palm on the body and the fingers toward the tail. He tests the motility capacity of the pancreas. Staying in this position, the osteopath can place one hand on the pancreas and another on the spleen where, toward the end of the movement of the pancreas, he should be able to feel a surge as both embryological movements are expressed within the same plane (Fig. 7.6).

Motility dysfunction

The endocrine pancreas, under a motility dysfunction, is in an extension dysfunction state and is restricted in its quarter-circle movement to the left.

Normalization

Normalizing the motility of the endocrine pancreas is usually carried out in the natural direction. Its synchronism with the movement of the spleen can be considered, but the normalization technique must be selected according to the

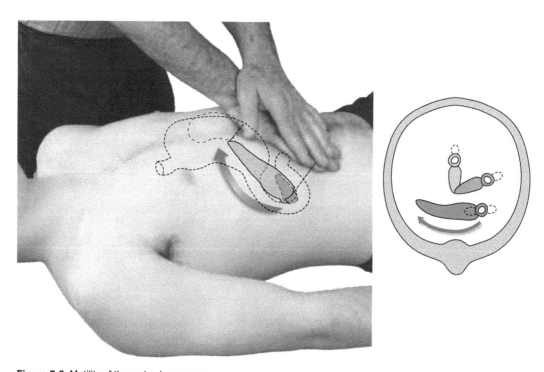

Figure 7.6. Motility of the endocrine pancreas.

characteristics of the dysfunction. An energy-deficiency dysfunction is an example of the type of dysfunction that might occur in the endocrine pancreas.

Links with traditional Chinese medicine

When associated with an emotion, dysfunctions of the endocrine pancreas can be linked to withdrawal into onself or a lack of the sense of self. The endocrine pancreas can therefore be affected by a motility dysfunction when personal space is not respected.

Osteopathic considerations

Lifting dysfunctions limiting the endocrine function of the pancreas helps to ensure proper insulin function. These pancreatic dysfunctions are usually significant. Normalizing these restrictions can sometimes cause hypoglycemic discomfort when insulin release is eased and happens too suddenly. The osteopath must take this into account in his clinical intervention.

Small intestine

Made up of two parts, the jejunum and the ileum, the small intestine plays many roles, the most significant being the absorption and assimilation of nutrients, and its involvement in immunity via Peyer's patches. Functionally and because of the direction of the movements, the second part of duodenum is continuous with the small intestine.

Embryological movement

The small intestine develops from the midgut. Initially, the midgut is a very small region between the anterior and posterior parts of the primitive gut, facing the yolk sac and umbilicus.

In the first stage of development, the small intestine develops around the superior mesenteric artery and since it elongates faster than the coelomic cavity, the primary intestinal loop develops in the extracoelomic space. Its proximal part will form the small intestine, while its distal part will form the colons.

The intestinal loop does a 90-degree counter-clockwise rotation around its longitudinal axis. The jejunum and ileum continue their rapid development by forming a series of folds. The intestinal loops are then reintegrated inside the abdominal cavity. This reintegration movement brings the small intestine from its sagittal position to a frontal position while pressing it against the posterior wall.

Motility movement and test

The small intestine's flexion motility movement is a counter-clockwise rotation around the superior mesenteric artery.

To evaluate the small intestine's motility, the osteopath places his hands obliquely on the inframesenteric region of the small intestine, along the mesenteric root orientation, and evaluates the small intestine's motility capacity (Fig. 7.7).

Motility dysfunction

The small intestine, under a motility loss, is in an extension dysfunction state and its normal movement is restricted in either one of its parts or in the whole organ.

Normalization

Normalizing the small intestine's motility is usually carried out in the natural direction (induction), but the normalization technique must be selected according to the characteristics of the dysfunction. An energy-deficiency dysfunction is an example of the type of dysfunction that might occur in the small intestine.

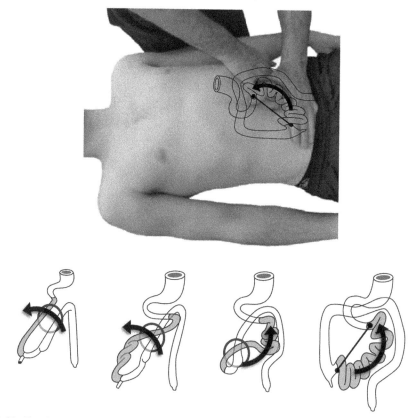

Figure 7.7. Motility of the small intestine.

Links with traditional Chinese medicine

When associated with an emotion, dysfunctions of the small intestine are, like the heart, linked to joy or the absence of joy.

Osteopathic considerations

Link with the assimilation of nutrients

Motility of the small intestine is essential to an optimal assimilation of nutrients; dysfunctions can lead to nutritional deficiency. The small intestine therefore plays a primary role in general health and in the production of the energy that fuels the organism's functions.

Link with the immune function

Via the Peyer's patches, the small intestine plays an important immune role. This capacity can be hindered by a motility and/or mobility dysfunction.

Links with the mesenteric root

An excess of tension in the mesenteric root can cause secondary dysfunctions of the sacroiliac joint to the right, in L2 to the left or in the duodenum via the ligament of Treitz. The mesenteric root will be much easier to treat if the small intestine's motility is normal.

Link with abdominal pressure

When there is an increase in general pressure in the abdomen, an osteopathic evaluation must distinguish, among the possible causes, the congestion of the small intestine secondary to a hepatic congestion overloading the portal venous system.

Colon

The colon's main roles are the storage of feces before they are excreted and the reabsorption of water and certain vitamins.

Embryological movement

The colon develops from the midgut and the hindgut.

The primary intestinal loop does a 90-degree counter-clockwise rotation around the superior mesenteric artery, which moves the cecum above the axis. It will then reintegrate the coelomic cavity by going from the sagittal to the frontal plane. During the change of plane, the cecum is moved under the liver. The counter-clockwise rotational growth of the ascending colon leads

the cecum into the right iliac fossa. At the same time, the distal part of the colon moves laterally to the left around the inferior mesenteric artery. From its central position, the sigmoid colon moves to the left. It will be attached to the wall by the two mesosigmoid roots (primary and secondary).

The ascending and descending colons are pressed against the posterior wall by the right and left Toldt's fasciae. The transverse colon is formed between the two.

The rectum develops from the distal part of the hindgut. The cloacal membrane opens at the seventh week, forming the anus and the urogenital system's orifices.

Motility movement and test

The colon's flexion motility movement is a counter-clockwise general movement. Its motility and transit movements are inverted.

To evaluate the colon's global motility, the osteopath may place his hands on the right and left colons and evaluate the colon's general motility capacity (Fig. 7.8).

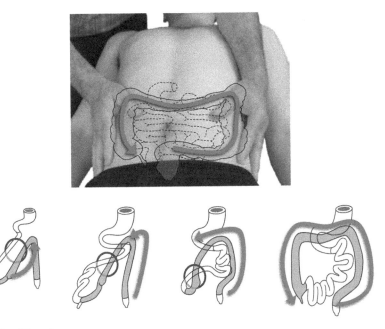

Figure 7.8. Motility of the colon.

To evaluate the specific motility of each part of the colon, the osteopath can successively move his hands during the evaluation. Starting at the sigmoid (Fig. 7.9A), he moves to the descending colon (Fig. 7.9B), then to the left colic flexure at the ninth rib and the left part of the transverse colon (Fig. 7.9C), then to the right part of the transverse colon and the right colic flexure at the 11th rib (7.9D), then to the ascending colon (Fig. 7.9E) and he finishes with the terminal part of the ascending colon and the cecum (Fig. 7.9F). He evaluates each part of the colon's motility capacity.

The rectum's motility is evaluated with the sacral plication. The osteopath looks for an upward movement parallel to the sacrum and for the rectum's motility capacity (for the corresponding positioning see the section on the caudal plication in Chapter 3).

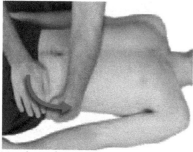

Motility of the sigmoid

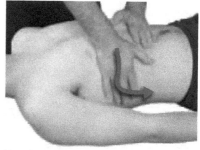

Motility of the right colic flexure and transverse colon

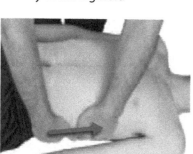

Motility of the descending colon

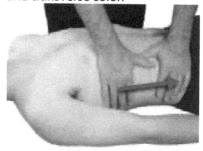

Motility of the ascending colon

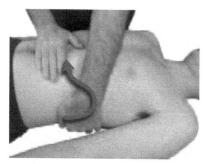

Motility of the left colic flexure and transverse colon

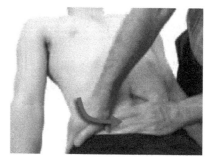

Motility of the ascending colon and caecum

Figure 7.9. Specific motility of the parts of the colon.
A. Motility of the sigmoid. **B.** Motility of the descending colon. **C.** Motility of the left colic flexure and transverse colon.
D. Motility of the right colic flexure and transverse colon. **E.** Motility of the ascending colon. **F.** Motility of the ascending colon and cecum.

Motility dysfunction

The colon, under a motility loss, is in an extension dysfunction state and is restricted in the normal movement of one of its parts or in its whole normal movement.

Embryological motility provides interesting explanations for the frequency of some of the colon's mobility dysfunctions. In addition to the quality of the system of tissular attachments of both colic flexures (better on the left and looser on the right), the embryological establishing movements can explain the rarity of ptosis in the left flexure and its higher rate of occurrence in the right flexure. In fact, embryological movements establish the left colic flexure from bottom to top, limiting the downward effect, but they establish the right colic flexure from top to bottom, enabling the downward effect. The upward motility movement of the rectum protects it from ptosis.

Normalization

Normalizing the colon's motility is usually carried out in the natural direction (induction), but the normalization technique must be selected according to the characteristics of the dysfunction. An energy-deficiency dysfunction is an example of the type of dysfunction that might occur in the colon.

The colon's various anatomic configurations and the specific characteristics of each of its parts call for specific treatments rather than a global approach.

Links with traditional Chinese medicine

When associated with an emotion, the dysfunctions of the colon affect only one side, and can be linked, like the lungs, to sadness. Therefore, considering the right and left colon separately, and their relation with the lung of the same side might be of interest.

When all of the colon's parts are under a motility dysfunction, it may be related to a difficult season change happening in the fall, which is a Chinese medicine concept.

Osteopathic considerations

Links with digestive function

Many reflexes, such as the gastrocolic reflex, regulate bolus transit in the colon. When the stomach fills, this reflex starts a mass movement that allows the transit of feces in the left part of the transverse colon, the descending colon and the sigmoid colon, filling the rectum. A hindered reflex might cause an atonic colon and constipation, but an increased reflex is more likely to cause too frequent excretion of feces. This increase in the gastrocolic reflex can be caused, for example, by a feeling of anxiety that affects the functioning of the the stomach.

Link with pathology

An intussusception (or invagination) is a dangerous and painful phenomenon occurring when a part of the intestine or colon is invaginated into an adjacent section. It occurs mostly in the ileocecal region in children under two years old, and especially between three and nine months old, but it can occur at any age. In 90 per cent of cases, the cause of intussusception is idiopathic (Williams 2008).

A dysfunctional schema involving an extension dysfunction of the small intestine when the cecum's motility is normal (the case of an ileocecal invagination) seems to indicate this type of invagination. The same principle can be applied for all forms of intussusception. Surgery can be avoided if the affected area is treated early enough with the correct osteopathic intervention. Note that, for reasons unknown, the frequency of this pediatric pathology seems to increase at the end of spring and in the fall, at least in Great Britain (Williams 2008). Could Chinese medicine provide an interpretation for this seasonal frequency (Fig. 7.10)?

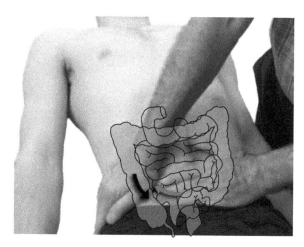

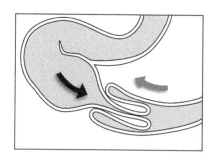

Figure 7.10. Intussusception.

References

Bonaz B (2010) Communication entre cerveau et intestin. La Revue de Médecine Interne 31, May 581–585.

Grundy D (2002) Neuroanatomy of visceral nociception: vagal and splanchnic afferent. Gut 51 i2–i5.

Guibert A and Guibert C (1973) Schémas d'anatomie du système nerveux central. Nerfs crâniens. Étude anatomo-clinique. Paris: Maloine.

Korr I M (1996) Bases physiologiques de l'ostéopathie. 2e édition. Frison-Roche.

Marieb E N (2005) Anatomie et physiologie humaines. Montréal: Editions du renouveau pédagogique.

Matricon J, Gelot A and Ardid D (2010) Mécanismes périphériques et centraux de l'hypersensibilité viscérale. Douleurs Évaluation – Diagnostic – Traitement 11 (2) April 65–74.

Nason K S, Wichienkuer P P, Awais O, Schuchert M J, Luketich J D, O'Rourke R W, Hunter J G, Morris C D and Jobe B A (2011) Gastroesophageal reflux disease symptom severity, proton pump inhibitor use, and esophageal carcinogenesis. Arch Surg 146 (7) July 851–858.

Régent D, Laurent V, Meyer-Bisch L, Barbary-Lefèvre C, Corby-Ciprian S and Mathias J (2006) La douleur biliaire : comment la reconnaître? comment l'explorer? J Radiol 87 413–429.

Verne G N, Robinson M E and Price D D (2001) Hypersensitivity to visceral and cutaneous pain in the irritable bowel syndrome. Pain 93 (1) July 7–14.

Williams H (2008) Imaging and intussusception. Arch Dis Child Ed Pract 93 (1) February 30–36.

Yamada T, Alpers D H, Laine L, Kaplowitz N, Owywang C and Poweel D W (2003) Yamada's Textbook of Gastroenterology. 4th edn. Philadelphia: Lippincott Williams & Wilkins.

Chapter 8

Urogenital System

Summary

This chapter focuses on the dysfunctions, tests, and normalizations for two systems that play very different roles despite being embryologically linked. In fact, although they are formed from similar common tubular structures containing the precursors of the urinary and reproductive systems, the two systems have very different functions. Clinically, the uterus and bladder are the most closely related, because their embryological movements are coordinated.

The kidney, ureter, and bladder are the elements to consider for the urinary system. Dysfunctions of the kidney are the most frequent, and their clinical consequences are varied.

The uterus is the most important element of the reproductive system, but the gonads are also frequently considered in motility work.

Interventions for the organs of the lesser pelvis are of course more common for women, with varied and sometimes disabling reasons for consultation including irregular menstrual cycle, congestion of the lesser pelvis and lower limbs, lumbosacral pains or pains pertaining to sexual intercourse, bladder incontinence, etc. Visceral motility work, often paired with work on the caudal plication, provides original solutions for these problems. For men, urogenital work is essentially aimed at prostate dysfunctions.

Dysfunctions of the kidney are frequently found in clinical practice and their effects are well-known to classical osteopathy, whether related to the vertebral column, the pelvis and the lower limbs, or to referred pain in the lower limbs caused by an irritation of the branches of the lumbosacral plexus. Because of its role in controlling arterial pressure, dysfunctions of the kidney can affect this important aspect of health. There are many reasons for dysfunctions. Dysfunctions of the kidney might have a structural cause such as loss of the layer of fat around the kidney due to rapid weight loss, a physical cause such as a trauma, or an emotional cause such as fear or failure to adapt to climatic changes.

Embryological generalities

The urogenital system develops from the intermediate mesoblast, with the exception of the bladder which is derived from the cloacal region of the hindgut. The parts of the urogenital system are either retroperitoneal (kidney and ureter) or infraperitoneal (genital organs and bladder).

The genital system, formed from the same tubular structures in both men and women, is completely integrated within the development of the urinary system. These structures are not described here as they are not related to the clinically useful embryological movements.

Urology

Kidney

The kidney ensures the essential functions of the human organism. Its main function is an exocrine function (blood filtration and urine excretion). It plays a role in the elimination of toxins – both endogenous toxins, such as the products of cellular senescence, and exogenous toxins, such as, for example, those associated with medication. The kidney also has an endocrine function in that it produces certain hormones: renin and kallikrein, which are related to the physiology of arterial pressure; and erythropoietin, which is related to the maturation of red blood cells in bone marrow. Therefore, the kidney takes part in homeostasis by maintaining the hydric, hydroelectrolytic, and acid-base equilibria.

Mechanically, its retroperitoneal position and a weak resistance to ptosis make the kidney very vulnerable to frequent mobility dysfunctions. The kidney depends on a layer of fat holding it in position, on the tonus of the abdominal muscles pressing it against the posterior wall, and on diaphragmatic aspiration, linked to a negative thoracic pressure, to help it resist ptosis. The upward movement of its motility is another protection factor against ptosis.

Embryological movement

The kidney is formed in three successive steps which lead to its final position. The two first iterations of the kidney go from a cephalic position to a caudal position. The definitive kidney (third iteration) is formed in the lesser pelvis before ascending to its dorsolumbar definitive position.

The **first kidney** is the pronephros and it forms at the level of the cervicodorsal junction. This metamerized kidney is present between the third and fourth week of embryonic life and regresses afterwards.

In the fourth week of embryonic life, the first kidney is replaced by the **second kidney**, which appears as a succession of metamerized mesonephros developing in a craniocaudal direction, the upper ones regressing as the lower ones are formed. This phenomenon starts from the cervicodorsal junction and ends in the lumbar region. Even if these temporary kidneys are never functional, they are connected to the cloaca by the Wolffian duct (or mesonephric duct). Starting from the eighth week, the mesonephros also begins to regress.

At the end of the fourth week, the metanephros, or **third kidney**, starts growing at sacral level S1–S3 from the ureteric bud located in the distal part of the Wolffian duct. From this rather caudal part of the embryo, the kidney, between the sixth and ninth weeks, progressively ascends up the dorsal aorta that ensures its vascularization with an array of arteries that emerge and regress following the upward movement. The kidney's ascent is caused by the differential growth of the caudal part of the embryo, described as the unwinding of the inferior part of the body (Drews 1994, p. 238). The movement happens toward the posterior wall and also includes an internal rotation. Indeed, the renal hilum, front-facing in the lesser pelvis, rotates 90 degrees to a medial direction in its definitive position (this rotation is properly illustrated in Cochard 2015, p. 163). The kidney's ascent causes a proportional elongation of the ureters.

The definitive kidney is formed between the fifth and 15th weeks of life. It is not metamerized. The height of the kidney's definitive position may vary significantly from one individual to another.

There are therefore two embryological movements to consider when evaluating the kidney's motility. The evaluation usually begins with the definitive (third) kidney's movement, which passes from the lesser pelvis to the lumbar region. If the treatment of the definitive kidney takes a long time or if pains at the level of the cervicodorsal junction imply motility dysfunctions of the first kidney, the evaluation will be completed by tests pertaining to the first and second kidneys.

Motility movement of the definitive kidney and test

The kidney's normal motility movement is an upward movement and an internal rotation.

To evaluate the kidney's motility, the osteopath begins his evaluation at the initial position of the definitive kidney (the lesser pelvis) and tests the kidney's motility capacity, first by evaluating the ascent capacity and then by evaluating the internal rotation capacity toward the definitive position. The kidney might be under a motility loss in either one of its movement's components or in both.

To perform this test, the osteopath can set a deep contact point near the kidney itself or stay on the surface at the Jarricot reflex zone, aiming for a proper visualization of the kidney and its movement while performing the test (Fig. 8.1).

He evaluates the motility movement from the cephalic point to the caudal point (Fig. 8.2).

Motility dysfunction

The definitive kidney, under a motility loss, is in an extension dysfunction state and is restricted in its upward movement and/or internal rotation movement.

Motility dysfunction

The two primitive kidneys, under a motility dysfunction, are in an extension dysfunction state and are restricted in their downward movement along the vertebral column.

Normalization

Normalizing the definitive kidney is carried out in the natural direction (induction).

Normalization

Normalizing the motility of the first and second kidneys is carried out in the natural direction (induction).

Motility movement of the first and second kidneys and test

The osteopath can also evaluate the energetic component of the successive movements of the first and second kidneys by evaluating motility along the column representing these movements. He places one hand at the cervicodorsal junction and the other on the inferior part of the kidney.

Links with traditional Chinese medicine

The kidney has a complex and fundamental place in Chinese medicine. Some basic considerations are presented here and, while they do not reflect the great significance of the kidney for traditional Chinese medicine, they point to important clinical elements.

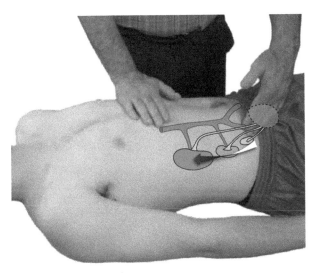

Figure 8.1. Motility of the definitive kidney.

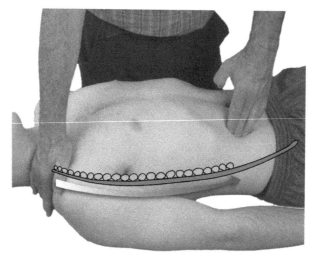

Figure 8.2. Motility of the first and second kidneys.

A primordial point of the kidney is located at the first dorsal vertebra, the Dazhu (Great Shuttle). Connections can be established between the primitive kidney (pronephros) and some recurrent pains at this location. The successive movements of the second kidney are resonant of the formation of part of the bladder meridian, along the vertebral column from top to bottom.

The kidney's role is different according to its laterality. The right kidney is linked to the feeling of too cold or too hot temperatures, and to drastic climatic changes. The left kidney is home to the fears of an individual, such as the fear of death or ancestral fears stored as engrams.

Finally, the kidney is linked to genetic energy and heredity.

Osteopathic considerations

The specific effects of a motility loss in the kidney almost always include a psoas reaction and often cause pains in the iliac crest on the side of the dysfunction. As previously stated, intractable dysfunctions of the cervicodorsal junction, linked to the primitive kidney, can also be found.

A kidney dysfunction can hinder the motility capacity of the caudalplication on the side of the affected kidney.

The effects of renal mobility dysfunctions, which are well-known to general osteopathy and are not listed here, also usually apply in the case of motility dysfunctions, taking into account the aforementioned distinctive features of this type of work, such as, for example, the usual primacy of motility dysfunctions over mobility dysfunctions.

Bladder

The bladder stores urine, received via the ureters before its excretion (urination) via the urethra. It usually contains between 300 and 700 milliliters of fluid. Normal relations with its environment are essential for the bladder to maintain its normal physiology, ensuring, depending on the time, its complete emptying and continence.

To ensure continence, the bladder benefits from two elements that 'suspend' it in the lesser pelvis. The first one is the upward imprint of its motility movement, which protects the bladder from ptosis at all times. To resist the increases in abdominal pressure that occur during maximum diaphragmatic inspiration, the bladder is also pulled upward by tension in the urachus and the falciform ligament caused by the posterior tilt of the liver associated with deep inspiration.

When it is properly 'suspended' in the lesser pelvis, abdominal pressure applies a compression force on the bladder, holding it and helping ensure the continence of the ureter's sphincter.

The length of the ureter subject to abdominal pressure and the different arrangement of its sphincters according to gender explain the significantly lower prevalence of incontinence disorders in men compared to women; incontinence disorders in men are most likely to be a sequela of surgery.

Proper functioning of the bladder is ensured by support from the pelvic floor and perineum, the functional integrity of the pelvic ring, and the capacity of the obturator membranes to act as valves. Functional deficiencies of the aforementioned 'suspension' structures of the bladder, or a surge of the uterus directly over it, can increase the workload of the sphincters and damage them over time causing stress incontinence or even, in severe cases, rest incontinence.

Significant dysfunctions, for example adhesions following an episiotomy, can locally hinder continence. In such cases, a local intervention and a prescription of short-term exercises for the striated sphincter (Kegel) usually succeed in getting rid of the problem. Such local problems must be distinguished from their counterparts involving the whole lesser pelvis region.

The causes of incontinence disorders are various and not all are mechanical. They can be of a hormonal nature given the role of hormones in the tissular tonus of the bladder and in its ligament support system; for example, incontinence often occurs during menopause.

The functioning of the bladder sphincters is also ensured by proper neural control. Control of the striated sphincter is ensured by the cortex. Control of the smooth sphincter is ensured by an orthosympathetic center located at upper lumbar level L1–L2; orthosympathetic information reaches the periphery through the celiac plexus.

Embryological movement

The bladder is derived from the cloacal region of the hindgut. At first, the bladder is a small diverticulum connected to the umbilicus, the allantois, sharing a common space with the distal part of the hindgut, the cloaca. The remnants of the allantois will form the urachus, or median umbilical ligament, in the definitive human body.

Between the fourth and sixth weeks, the descent of the urorectal septum splits the cloaca into two structures, the urogenital sinus and the anorectal canal, that will connect to the exterior via two distinct orifices.

The ducts forming the ureters open in the bladder and help form the trigone of the bladder in its posterior wall.

The bladder's movement, in going through these iterations toward its definitive position, is a slight ascent at first, followed by a posterior rotation.

Motility movement and test

The bladder's normal motility movement is a slight upward movement and a posterior rotation.

To evaluate the bladder's motility, the osteopath places his fingers in the crease just above the pubic symphysis and tests the bladder's motility capacity.

To test the bladder's mobility, the osteopath stays in the same position and asks the subject to breathe in and out deeply in order to feel the pull of the urachus during inspiration and its easing during expiration. This information complements the evaluation of motility.

The bladder's motility is also considered in its synchronism with the caudal plication, which may seem disrupted when the bladder is affected by a dysfunction. Depending on the reason for consultation, the synchronism of the bladder's motility with that of the uterus may need to be tested (Fig. 8.3).

Motility dysfunction

The bladder, under a motility loss, is in an extension dysfunction state and is restricted in its upward and posterior rotation movements.

A bladder dysfunction can hinder the motility of the caudal plication in its central part.

Normalization

Normalizing the bladder's motility is carried out in the natural direction (induction), or according

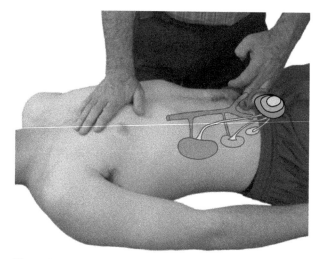

Figure 8.3. Motility of the bladder.

to characteristics of the dysfunction. It is completed by checking for synchronism with the caudal plication and, in some cases, with the uterus.

A bladder dysfunction, especially an energy-deficiency dysfunction combined with a dysfunction of the caudal plication (which is hard to lift even after a proper treatment), might indicate bladder cancer, often caused by smoking (see Clinical case 20 in Chapter 10).

Links with traditional Chinese medicine

When associated with an emotion, dysfunctions of the bladder are linked to a very intense fear that 'overflowed' to the bladder. The 'climatic' kidney may sometimes be the cause of this phenomenon.

Osteopathic considerations

Continence

Motility's specific contribution to urinary continence is the embryological movement's upward direction that protects the bladder from ptosis.

Links with cystitis

Correct posterior tilt motility allows for a proper orientation of the urethra. An improper orientation may prevent the complete emptying of the bladder during urination. Urine stagnation caused by this condition obviously leads to recurring urinary infections. Other elements must be considered such as the functioning of the liver and small intestine as their circulatory and immune roles may be related to the onset of cystitis. Nutrition must also be considered as it has a considerable impact on the body's pH control mechanisms. In the case of recurrent cystitis, it is useful to distinguish the type of bacteria, to get rid of fever, and to consider the passage of pathogens through the adjacent walls of the bladder and small intestine. In such cases, the dysfunction of the digestive system must be treated first.

Vesicoureteral reflux

Vesicoureteral reflux to the kidney can cause hydronephrosis. Occurring when the sphincter between the ureter and bladder is ineffective, it can sometimes affect children. Some cases of vesicoureteral reflux or hydronephrosis are 'osteopathic' and can be treated with precise osteopathic normalizations of the links between the kidneys, ureter, and bladder.

Enuresis

Enuresis can be related to the reticular formation if urination is controlled during the day but not at night. The first thing to test is therefore the posterior wall of the first fold followed by evaluation of the celiac plexus that ensures the sphincter's innervation.

Ureters

The ureter's movement is secondary to the movement of the kidneys and bladder. The progressive elongation of the ureter is induced by the kidney's upward movement. The ureter also rotates internally along all of its length, this movement being induced by both the kidney's internal rotation and the bladder's posterior rotation. The ureter's normal motility is therefore deduced from the motility capacity of the kidney and bladder.

Synchronism of the movement of the ureters with the bladder's posterior tilt movement is essential to preventing vesicoureteral refluxes. Such refluxes can sometimes be explained by osteopathy; they are then regulated by motility work. This type of reflux must be distinguished from a structural reflux, which can be explained by allopathic medicine.

Following episodes of renal colic, tension zones can appear in the ureter, which will eventually affect the homolateral kidney. These tensions will be easier to regulate using local mobility techniques once the ureter has recovered its energetic movement and its synchronism with the kidney and bladder (Fig. 8.4).

Genital organs

Embryological generalities

The genital system, formed from the same tubular structures in men and women, is completely integrated with the development of the urinary system.

Before sexual differentiation of the embryo, two pairs of ducts pertaining to the kidney's development are found: the Wolffian ducts (or mesonephric ducts), important to the male reproductive organs, and the Müllerian ducts (paramesonephric ducts), important to the female reproductive organs. In males, Wolffian ducts develop into the ductus deferens, while the Müllerian ducts atrophy. In females, the Müllerian ducts develop into the uterus and the upper part of the vagina where they fuse (the lower part is formed by the endoderm), and they also form

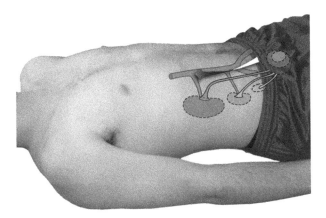

Figure 8.4. Motility of the ureter.

both Fallopian tubes. The Wolffian ducts atrophy and disappear almost completely in females.

Uterus

The uterus is a hollow organ of which the primary role is to house and nurture the fertilized ovum. Its smooth muscles allow for the expulsion of the baby during childbirth with powerful and rhythmic contractions.

The uterus is protected from abdominal pressure by its position in the pelvic outlet.

Embryological movement

Both Müllerian ducts fuse to form one cavity. The definitive position and form of the uterus is achieved following an upward movement and an anterior rotation, the opposite of the bladder's movement, which is located just in front and below the uterus.

Motility movement and test

The normal motility movement of the uterus is an upward movement and an anterior rotation.

To evaluate the motility of the uterus, the osteopath places one hand on the sacrum, in the same position as for the caudal plication test, and places the other hand on the uterus just above the pubis. He tests the motility capacity of the uterus and also checks the synchronicity of the movement with movements of the caudal plication and bladder (Fig. 8.5).

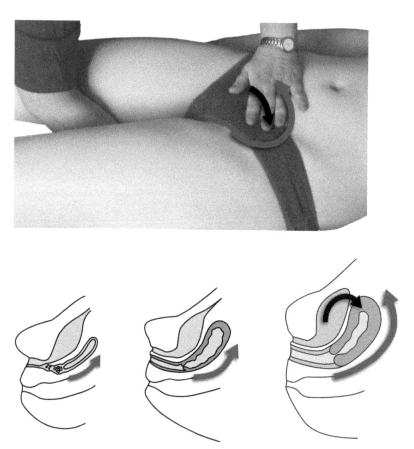

Figure 8.5. Motility of the uterus.

Motility dysfunction

The uterus, under a motility dysfunction, is in an extension dysfunction state and is restricted in its upward and anterior rotation movements. The osteopath then does not feel a surge under his anterior hand but he can feel a disruption in the perception of the caudal plication's motility. Energy deficiency dysfunctions of the uterus are possible but scarce.

Normalization

Normalizing the uterus is carried out with indirect techniques (accumulation). It is completed by looking for synchronism with the caudal plication, and, in some cases, with the bladder.

Normalizing a uterine dysfunction with natural direction techniques (induction) can be carried out by placing one hand directly at the uterine cervix, in the anterior cul-de-sac (or excavatio vesicouterina), to induce flexion motility with a direct contact point.

Links with traditional Chinese medicine

The uterus, given its muscular nature, can be influenced by the energetic function of the pericardium meridian and by the energetic function of the liver.

Osteopathic considerations

When faced with dysmenorrhea, both the production and diffusion capacities of the hypothalamic–pituitary axis and the hormone reception capacities of the target organs (uterus and ovaries) must be checked. Freedom of the lesser pelvis region must be sufficient enough to ensure the proper transport of hormones through its essential circulatory axis.

Amenorrhea of an 'osteopathic' origin, unrelated to the general state of health, requires an investigation of the superior commands: the condition will be resolved by work on the central nervous system and on the hypothalamic–pituitary axis rather than local work.

Dyspareunia of a mechanical rather than emotional origin is usually related to local mobility and motility disorders; it is treated by finding and normalizing the restrictions.

The first step in infertility cases is to check the freedom of the uterine tubes. Then, according to the context, the necessary local normalizations are performed for a proper motility and mobility of the reproductive organs. It is also essential that a suitable environment is ensured through regulation of the caudal plication and by allowing correct vascularization via optimal functioning of the celiac and hypogastric plexuses. Furthermore, the autonomous nervous system must be considered, and the first and third fold evaluated and normalized.

Gonads: ovaries and testicles

Containing the germ cells, the ovaries and testicles are essential to genetic transmission.

Embryological movement

The gonads are the first parts of the reproductive system that develop from the genital ridges which are linked to the upper wall by the cranial suspensory ligament and to the lower wall by the gubernaculum. In females, the superior part remains and becomes the suspensory ligament of the ovary – also containing the ovarian arteries – while the medial part becomes the utero-ovarian ligament and the inferior part becomes the round ligament.

In males, the inferior part remains and guides the testicles' descent, while the superior part of the ligament disappears.

When ready to host them, the gonads receive the germ cells that were, up to this point, contained in the yolk sac.

Motility movement and test

The normal motility movement of the ovaries and testicles is a descent and an external rotation.

To evaluate the motility of the ovaries and testicles, the osteopath places his hands at the starting point of the ovaries' descent, slightly around the umbilicus (under the renal arteries) and tests the motility capacity of the ovaries (or testicles) (Fig. 8.6).

Motility dysfunction

The ovary or testicle, under a motility loss, is in an extension dysfunction state and is restricted in its downward and external rotation movements.

A key element in confirming an ovarian dysfunction would be the difficulty a woman has in lifting her pelvis while lying on her back.

Normalization

Normalizing motility of the ovaries or testicles is usually carried out in the natural direction (induction).

Osteopathic considerations

For ovaries

'Functional' ovarian cysts, different from structural cysts of an embryological, tumoral, etc. origin, can be linked to energetic dysfunctions of the ovaries, of which the mobility should also be tested. Dysfunctions of the hypothalamic–pituitary axis must also be considered.

For testicles

In cases of improper testicular descent, the L1 level must be investigated as it is the neurological control of the cremasteric reflex and cremaster muscles. The testicles' motility should also be verified.

Recurrent epididymitis is also often linked to the L1 level. It can therefore be linked to energetic dysfunctions of the stomach.

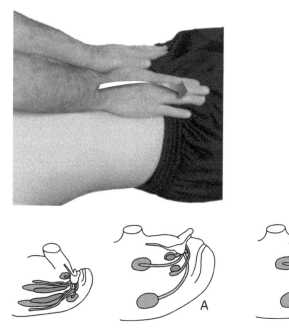

Figure 8.6. Motility of the gonads: male **(A)** and female **(B)** development.

Prostate

The prostate wraps around the urethra. It is a male genital gland that secretes and stores part of the seminal fluid. Its weight increases from birth and stabilizes around adolescence. In the forties, its volume and weight may increase again. In some older subjects, the prostate is sometimes hypertrophic, possibly achieving sizes seven times larger than the size at puberty. It then hinders urination, limiting its flow and increasing its frequency.

In this work, the prostate is an exception because it develops in its definitive position, and therefore its embryological movement is fairly limited. The very small upward movement is essentially the result of growth of its vertical diameter. This small upward movement is the one to evaluate. To ensure the prostate's normal functions, the bladder's proper upward movement is essential to avoid compression.

Motility movement and test

The prostate's normal motility movement is a short ascent.

To evaluate the prostate's motility, the osteopath places one hand on the sacrum (same position as for the caudal plication test) and the other on the prostate, just above the pubis. He tests the prostate's motility capacity, taking into account the possible restrictions of the bladder.

Motility dysfunction

The prostate, under a motility loss, is in an extension dysfunction state and is restricted in its upward movement. The osteopath may feel a disruption in the perception of the caudal plication's motility. He can validate the results of energetic tests against the results of classical mobility tests.

Osteopathic considerations

Through neural and/or circulatory pathways, chronic prostatitis can be linked to sacrococcygeal dysfunctions.

References

Drews U (1994) Atlas de poche d'embryologie. Broché Flammarion Médecine-Sciences.

Cochard L R (2015) Atlas d'embryologie humaine de Netter Trans. Stéphane Louryan. De Boeck.

Chapter 9

Musculoskeletal System

Summary

This chapter focuses on disorders of the musculoskeletal system. Although these types of disorders are the most common reason for consulting an osteopath (Dubois & Coatmellec 2012, Orrock 2009, Fawkes et al. 2010, Morin & Aubin 2012), this, of course, does not mean that the primary causes lie in the musculoskeletal system. This chapter touches on explanations for chronic and/or recurring disorders affecting the musculoskeletal system. Embryological generalities are outlined first, followed by explanations of the motility dysfunctions and the tests and techniques for normalization of the vertebral column (both as a whole and in a segmental way), the ribs and spinal nerves, the scapular girdle and the upper limb, and finally the ilium and the lower limb. The use of motility techniques for the bones of the cranium bones is discussed at the end of the chapter.

Supporting the body, the musculoskeletal system is composed of connective tissue of varying density, bones, muscles, fasciae/aponeuroses and the deep layers of the skin. Since basic dysfunctions of this system are most likely to involve bones and joints (soft tissue disorders often being consequences of these dysfunctions), the descriptions presented here will be limited to the densest parts of the system, even though the specific applications could be considered for the connective tissue as well.

Local and recent affections of the musculoskeletal system, often caused by a trauma, can frequently be resolved with classic mobility techniques, but chronic pain, without a mechanical pain pattern or with atypical signs and symptoms, will benefit from the motility model of clinical interpretation because the real causes of constant vertebral or peripheral pain have to be located.

Recurring or chronic pain that is slow to heal completely for no obvious reason is often linked to compression factors, caused either by general tension of the dura mater – affecting the vertebral column and the lower limbs – or by tensions in the thoracic region – especially affecting the upper limbs. Local dysfunctions of the vertebral column and limbs can also be consequences of a long-standing motility disruption that causes devitalization. It is also essential to consider the numerous links with the visceral sphere when looking for the causal factors. Finally, chronic pain that resists classical techniques may be imprinted in the nervous system, which may explain its persistence (see Chapter 5).

Embryological generalities

Vertebral column and ribs

The development of the vertebral axis starts at the third week of pregnancy and is followed by the metamerization process of the nervous system and vertebral column that allows for the segmental organization of the embryo.

At day 20, the first structure of the vertical axis, the **notochord**, appears. It develops in a cephalic direction from the caudal end of the central axis (see Fig. 3.4). The notochord is essential to the development of the neural plate, which is in turn responsible for the development of vertebrae, but the only notochord part that subsists in the definitive body is the one that forms the nucleus pulposus in all intervertebral discs. During the fourth week of embryonic life, the neural plate progressively develops from the endoderm. It sinks while winding over on itself, forming a hollow tube (the neurulation process). The vertebrae develop from the mesoderm after the medulla is formed, since they wrap around and protect the latter in the definitive body.

From day 20 to day 30, the paraxial mesoderm is organized in **somites** (see Fig. 3.6) that are quickly subdivided into sclerotomes (which form vertebrae and ribs), myotomes (which form the striated muscles of the limbs and torso), and dermatomes (which form the subcutaneous tissue). The somites develop in the opposite direction to the notochord, from the cervical region to the sacrum (cephalocaudal direction). From 42–44 somites initially, the total number dwindles to 37 in the definitive body. The cephalic-most somites form the striated muscles of the face, jaw, and pharynx (pharyngeal arches), while the caudal-most ones disappear. The definitive organism contains four somites in the occipital region, eight cervical somites, 12 thoracic somites, five lumbar somites, five sacral somites and three coccygeal somites.

The developing **sclerotomes** wrap around the notochord and fill the perimeter of the neural tube from front to back. The body of the vertebra is therefore formed first, followed by the posterior arch. Then, the sclerotomes progressively densify. Three ossification centers are present in a vertebra from the ninth/tenth week until birth (body and two neural arches); the definitive vertebral ossification is completed at 25 years old.

Formation of each individual vertebra (resegmentation) happens around the 40th day, originating from the fusion of two segmental half-sclerotomes, the cranial half-sclerotome of an inferior somite and the caudal half-sclerotome of a superior somite. This particular disposition allows the spinal nerve's emergence between two vertebrae and its truly segmental nature. Resegmentation can explain why there are eight cervical spinal nerves for seven vertebral levels.

From the 35th day, **ribs** develop from small lateral mesenchymal condensations called costal processes at cervical and dorsal levels. The ribs are normally fully formed only at the dorsal level. The ribs help the lateral closure of the thorax by progressively elongating from the posterior wall toward the anterior junction with the sternum; the junction happens at the 45th day. The **sternum** is formed by the fusion of two sternal bars that join on the median line and fuse in the ninth week.

Limbs

The limb buds develop from the somatic mesoderm. The upper limb buds appear at the 26th day, two days before the lower limb buds. Each bud is covered in endoderm, which will form the superficial skin layer. At the fifth week, the limbs are called plates, because of their flattened shape. The regular shape of the limbs forms between the fourth and eighth weeks, during which time the limbs grow in the caudal direction. At the eighth week, the limbs are formed from three segments, with a fold in their medial segment forming the elbow or knee. A 90-degree rotation then occurs, external for the upper limb (moving the elbow in a posterior direction) and internal for the lower limb (moving the knee in an anterior direction). The limbs' rotations explain the definitive coiled shape of the dermatomes, because the branches of the brachial and lumbosacral nervous plexuses follow the rotational development of the limbs.

The **upper limb** bud is located around the six last cervical metameres and the two first dorsal metameres, and receives its innervation from these vertebral levels. It contains the mesodermal condensations that will form the scapula, humerus, radius, ulna, and all the bones of the carpus, the hands and the fingers. The collarbone develops at the anterior part of the thorax from a distinct ossification center that appears at the seventh week.

The **lower limb** bud is located around the four last lumbar metameres and the three first sacral metameres, and receives its innervation from these vertebral levels. It contains the mesodermal condensations that will form the pubis, ilium, femur, tibia, fibula, and all the bones of the feet and toes.

General vertebral column, notochord, and vertebral segments

Motility movement and test

To evaluate the **notochord's general motility**, the osteopath slides his hand along the vertebral column from bottom to top, focusing his attention on the nucleus pulposus of each disc. He checks for any disruption in this upward motility movement (Fig. 9.1).

To evaluate the **vertebral column's general motility**, the osteopath slides his hand along the vertebral column from top to bottom. A disruption in the downward movement hints at a segmental dysfunction. The osteopath can then go further by evaluating the density characteristics and the motility losses, and, eventually, the presence of mechanical vertebral osteopathic dysfunctions (Fig. 9.2).

To evaluate the **segmental motility of a vertebra**, the osteopath uses the articular processes as the contact point. He presses lightly and tests the return capacity. The motility movement to look for is the anteroposterior movement, associated with the movement of the articular process. Because of its direction, the testing of this movement calls for an indirect technique. Depending on the response, the

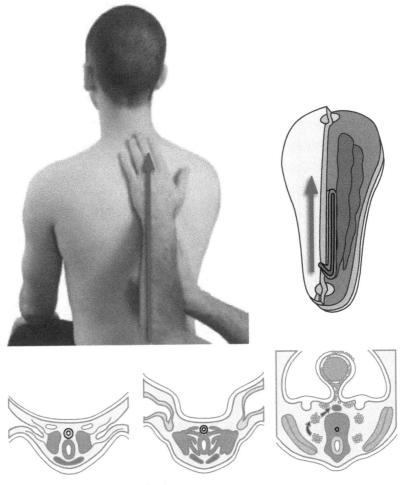

Figure 9.1. Motility of the notochord.

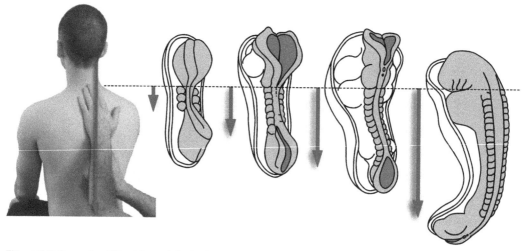

Figure 9.2. General motility of the vertebral column.

conclusion might point to a unilateral or bilateral dysfunction, or to a 'tripod' or 'translation' dysfunction, when there are associated costal dysfunctions and a proper clinical context (Fig. 9.3).

Furthermore, it is possible to evaluate the **motility of the roots of the spinal nerves**. The osteopath places one hand on each side of the vertebral level and evaluates the spinal nerve's flexion motility capacity in an outward direction. This movement is identical to the costal movement but pertains to the spinal nerve's own movement when detected between two ribs.

Motility dysfunction

The notochord, under a motility loss, is in an extension dysfunction state and is restricted in its upward movement.

The vertebral column, under a motility loss, is in an extension dysfunction state and is restricted in its downward movement.

The vertebral segment, under a motility loss, is in an extension dysfunction state and is restricted in its anteroposterior movement.

The spinal nerve, under a motility loss, is in an extension dysfunction state and is restricted in its outward movement.

Normalization

Normalizing the notochord's motility is usually carried out in the natural direction (induction).

Normalizing the vertebral column's motility is usually carried out in the natural direction (induction).

Normalizing a vertebral segment's motility is usually carried out with indirect techniques (accumulation).

Normalizing the spinal nerve's motility is usually carried out in the natural direction (induction).

Osteopathic considerations

Compressions affecting the vertebral column are usually linked to tensions of the spinal dura mater. In such cases, it is better to ensure the proper motility of the thoracic and caudal plications as well as that of the cranial folds before directly normalizing membranes or local vertebral dysfunctions. This general decompression work can be completed by the top-to-bottom energetic work on the vertebral column described above, even if the primary purpose of this movement's evaluation is to find the actual level of a segmental dysfunction.

This segmental vertebral work is also usually secondary to spinal cord and neural crest work (as

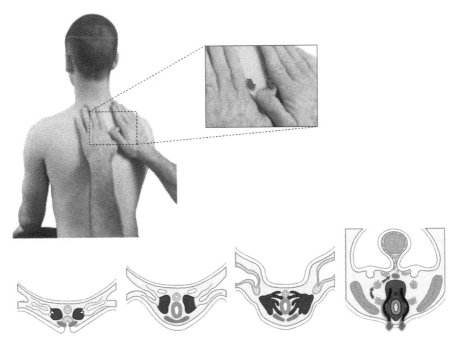

Figure 9.3. Segmental motility of the vertebrae.

described in Chapter 5), but it can still sometimes provide solutions to persisting vertebral problems.

Some recurring conflicts affecting spinal nerves can be caused by an energy differential between the notochord and the spinal cord at a precise point of the vertebral column. To treat such cases, the proper first step is to find the seemingly primary dysfunction, often signaled by a greater intensity, and to restore its proper motility; it is also essential to normalize the synchronism between the two movements. This work should be frequently completed by normalization of the motility of the spinal nerve and neural crest, and, sometimes, by mobility work since it would then be fully effective.

Ribs

Motility movement and test

The general development movement of the ribs starts from the vertebral column, in the direction of the sternum. The rib slightly rotates in the posterior direction, twisting around its axis,

when forming its anterior junction with the sternum.

To evaluate the rib's general motility, the osteopath places one hand below the posterior arch and another on the junction between the rib and the sternal cartilage. He can also, if possible, place one hand on the costal angle to feel the motility's passage from back to front.

The osteopath evaluates the rib's motility capacity (Fig. 9.4).

Motility dysfunction

The rib, under a motility loss, is in an extension dysfunction state and is restricted in its closure movement around the thorax and in its posterior rotation movement around its longitudinal axis. This restriction can be complete or partial, and can affect one or several of the movement's components.

Normalization

Normalizing the costal motility is usually carried out in the natural direction (induction).

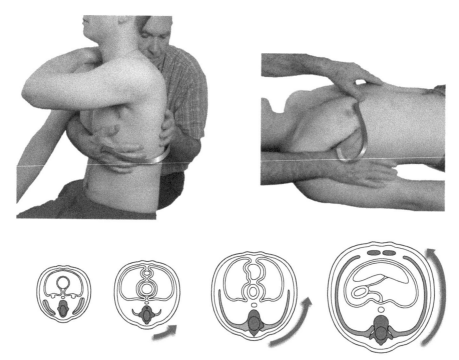

Figure 9.4. Motility of the ribs.

Osteopathic considerations

Isolated costal motility dysfunctions are quite rare. Costal motility dysfunctions are usually occur alongside vertebral dysfunctions, dysfunctions of the spinal nerve, or dysfunctions of the parietal pleura.

A severe costal dysfunction, located at a precise level, may favor the appearance of shingles if there is contact with the virus.

Upper limb

Motility movement and test

The upper limb develops in a caudal direction, performing an external global rotation that brings the elbow to the back.

To evaluate the motility of the scapula and collarbone, the osteopath places one hand on each bone and tests their outward movement (caudal movement), and then their posterior rotation movement (Fig. 9.5).

To evaluate the motility of the humerus and distal part of the upper limb, the osteopath places one hand on the upper part of the humerus and the other on the radius and ulna and tests their caudal movement, and then their external rotation movement. The evaluation is the same for the hand and fingers (Fig. 9.6).

Motility dysfunctions

The upper limb, under a motility loss, is in an extension dysfunction state and is restricted in its downward movement and/or external rotation movement.

Normalization

Normalizing the upper limb's motility is usually carried out in the natural direction (induction).

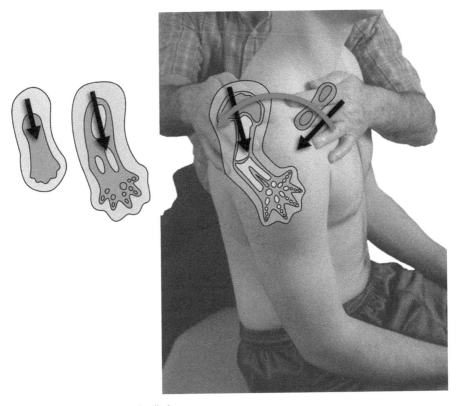

Figure 9.5. Motility of the scapula and collarbone.

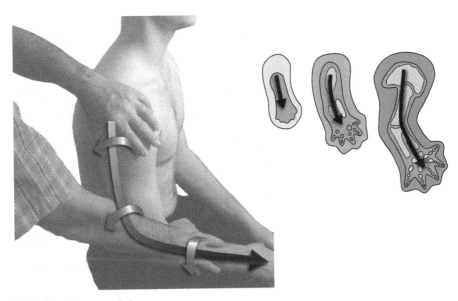

Figure 9.6. Motility of the upper limb.

Osteopathic considerations

Restrictions of the upper limb of the compression type are often secondary to blockages found in the thoracic region. When the upper limb loses its motility movement in the caudal direction, its joints are under an excess of tension in the direction of the compression, which hinders normal physiology and makes these joints more vulnerable to rotator cuff impingement or humeral head osteoarthritis. Tension can spread as far as the forearm, interosseous membrane and wrist, and it can be linked, for example, with carpal tunnel syndrome, which is caused by compression of the median nerve. Local normalizations are usually ineffective until the compressive factor affecting the upper limb is lifted.

Mechanical-rotation and counter-rotation factors may be present to counter the compression. They predispose to several pathologies of the soft tissues, which may lose their integrity when under this external coercion. Tendinitis, bursitis, etc., will, in such cases, appear without any underlying rational explanation.

Lower limb

Motility movement and test

The lower limb develops in a caudal direction, performing an internal global rotation that brings the knee to the front. To evaluate its general motility, the osteopath uses successive contact points along the lower limb.

To evaluate the general motility of the ilium, the osteopath places one hand on the iliac crest and the other on the lower limb. He tests the outward movement, associated with the caudal development of the lower limb, and then the internal rotation movement (Fig. 9.7).

To evaluate the general motility of the femur and distal part of the lower limb, the osteopath places one hand on the upper part of the femur and the other on the tibia and fibula. He tests the elongation movement and the internal rotation

movement. The evaluation is the same for the foot and toes (Fig. 9.8).

Motility dysfunction

The ilium, under a motility loss, is in an extension dysfunction state and is restricted in its outward movement and/or internal rotation movement.

The lower limb, under a motility loss, is in an extension dysfunction state and is restricted in its downward movement and/or internal rotation movement.

Normalization

Normalizing the motility of the ilium and lower limb is usually carried out in the natural direction (induction).

Osteopathic considerations

Restrictions of the lower limb of the compression type are often secondary to blockages found in the membranes of the craniosacral system.

When the lower limb loses its motility movement in the caudal direction, joints of the hip, knee and ankle, as well as the interosseous membrane, are under an excess of tension in the direction of the compression, hindering normal physiology. A long-lasting compressive factor predisposes to early osteoarthritis and explains why the latter can appear on only one of the joints of the lower limb. As for the upper limb – maybe even more so because they are load-bearing – the joints of the lower limb try to counter the compressive effect with mechanical rotation and counter-rotation movements that can cause several types of recurring or chronic musculoskeletal conditions affecting the soft tissues, such as bursitis or tendinitis. For the lower limb, too, local normalizations are usually ineffective until the compressive factor is properly lifted.

Even more so than for the upper limb, isolated dysfunctions are sometimes found at the femur or

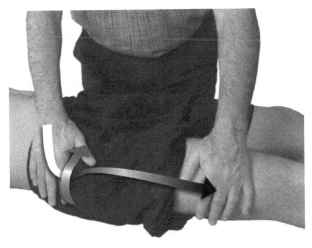

Figure 9.7. Motility of the ilium.

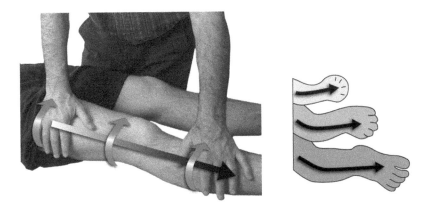

Figure 9.8. Motility of the lower limb.

tibia, without a compressive factor. They are then usually linked to development and they indicate misalignment, of which the effects appear during growth in children.

Cranial bones

Cranial bones, like any other structure of the body, have their own motility movement corresponding to their embryological development. There is no need to clinically describe all these motility movements since they depend on the nervous system's functions and therefore on its

motility, given the relationship between container and contents. Unlike the thoracic and abdominopelvic containers, the contents of the cranium are established before its container. This developmental primacy prevails until the definitive cranium is functioning.

Evaluating and normalizing motility dysfunctions of the central nervous system is thus the first step of cranial work. If dysfunctions of the bones or sutures persist after this work, they are usually likely to be successfully treated with classical cranial techniques.

Specifically normalizing the embryological movement of the facial bones may be clinically useful for some patients. Overall, this movement follows the general lateral inflection movement of the body, joining the left and right part of the facial bones on the central line. This plication movement must be distinguished from the facial bones' growth movement, which is a general downward movement.

References

Dubois T and Coatmellec J (2012) Osteopathy in France: A demographic and epidemiologic descriptive analysis of French osteopaths' patients. Paris: OIA.

Fawkes C, Leach J, Mathias S and Moore A P (2010) Standardised data collection within osteopathic practice in the UK: development and first use of a tool to profile osteopathic care in 2009. Clinical Research Centre for Health Professions, University of Brighton. National Council for Osteopathic Research (NCOR).

Morin C and Aubin A (2012) Survey on osteopathic practices in Quebec: Most common reasons for consultation. Paris: OIA.

Orrock P (2009) Profile of members of the Australian Osteopathic Association: Part 2 – The Patients. International Journal of Osteopathic Medicine 12 (4) December 128–139.

Chapter 10

Clinical Intervention Protocol for the Motility Model

The osteopathic approach implies a constant adaptation to the reason for consultation. Despite this necessity, elaborating the steps of an intervention protocol is useful to maximize its effectiveness, to guide the intentions and to organize the conclusions. The intervention protocol is not meant to include all the information needed or to illustrate all possible cases, especially in the descriptions of local interventions for the three spheres (cranial, visceral, musculoskeletal) where it is only representational, but can still be of help to the clinician who is trying to integrate the embryology-based motility concept into his therapeutic arsenal. Real clinical cases are described alongside the protocol, representing, each in their own way, what may be achieved with the application of motility techniques.

An important underlying principle of the intervention protocol is that it closely follows the sequences of embryonic development. It has been proved many times in clinical practice that respecting these sequences reduces the risk of an adverse or disproportionate reaction to energetic treatments.

The three first weeks of life are essentially dedicated to rapid growth in the number of cells and to their organization into a trilaminar disc around a vertical axis. No specific structures are developed at this point. The first step of the clinical intervention protocol begins with the evaluation and normalization of the thoracic and caudal plications which form in the fourth week of embryonic life. Because they establish the heart, diaphragm, and thoracic and abdominopelvic containers, the plications reflect the general organization of the body. This first step is usually followed by work on the folds of the neural tube, which form in the fourth and fifth embryonic week. Work on significant dysfunctions of the plexuses sometimes completes these first two interventions, although it does not strictly follow the embryological sequence of development.

These first three steps enable the therapist to rapidly assess the complexity of the case. Evaluating the plications and the central nervous system, which will also provide information on the plexuses, the diaphragm, and the dura mater, enables the therapist to recognize complex cases where the organism is under significant strain and the general adaptation capacity has possibly been reduced. In these situations, it is better to start with clinical interventions which aim to recover the body's adaptation capacity, which will in turn ensure more effective local normalizations.

After these steps, the protocol becomes more specific to the reason for the consultation and shifts toward a regional or local aspect of one of the three spheres (cranial, visceral, or musculoskeletal). A targeted evaluation, depending on the case, considers both the embryological development sequences and the circulation of neural information. This information can travel in a centripetal direction to the viscera, cranium, and musculoskeletal system by going from the central nervous system to the autonomous nervous system, the nuclei of the cranial nerves, the medulla oblongata, the spinal cord, the neural crests, and the ganglia, toward the plexuses and spinal nerves. In a centrifugal direction, the information can take various routes: the vagal and splanchnic pathways carry visceral information and they are closely related to the first fold of the neural tube.

Describing the pathways followed by information from the musculoskeletal system is not useful here, but they can sometimes be related to the sensory homunculus, which is an important clinical element of the embryology-based motility concept.

As with classical osteopathy, some reasons for consultation will be interpreted from a causal angle or from the container–contents relationship (cranial, thoracic, pelvic containers and their contents) point of view.

When the motility concept is mastered, it is almost always more useful to begin the intervention with motility techniques, and to complete it with mobility techniques (see Chapter 1). This principle is of course tailored to the characteristics of the dysfunctions and according to the appearance, development, and persistence of the signs and symptoms. During a clinical intervention, the experienced practitioner normalizes dysfunctions and blockages as he discovers them, especially when they can explain, in whole or in part, the reason for consultation.

The first three steps of the protocol

Thoracic and caudal plications

The first step of the protocol is always to evaluate the thoracic and caudal plications (Fig. 10.1), as they need to have sufficient motility before the osteopath proceeds any further with the clinical intervention. Dysfunctions of these plications, varying in intensity, are very frequent. Although it might seem vague at first, the 'sufficient' level become easier to determine as the osteopath learns by evaluating and normalizing a reasonable number of cases, which enables him to develop expertise.

The level of freedom of the plications gives an idea of the body's general vitality since this freedom illustrates an absence of compressions or significant hindrances to the axial and deep structures of the body and constitutes an essential condition for the proper movement of the diaphragm.

Clinical case 1

Normalizing the thoracic and caudal plications

Plications are not usually treated in isolation, but sometimes normalizing them can relieve the axial structures even if the structure is altered. This was the case for a patient in his late forties, who was suffering from ankylosing spondylitis and who had a fairly physical job as an antiques dealer. His posture was typical of this pathology: major postural modifications caused pain along the length of the vertebral column and hindered its mobility.

Normalizing the motility of the plications had substantially alleviated the pain for more than ten years (during a few sessions each year) by allowing the axial structure to retrieve better vitality despite significant mobility losses in the vertebral column, which had obviously remained.

Perception of the whole movement of the plications can be altered if significant dysfunctions are present in other structures. In this way, the movement of the thoracic plication may be hindered by dysfunctions of the fibrous pericardium or of the celiac and/or cardiopulmonary plexuses. The movement of the caudal plication may be hindered, on one side, by renal dysfunctions, which are quite frequent. In its central part, it can be hindered by dysfunctions of the uterus, the bladder or the rectum. It can also be hindered, on one side, by dysfunctions of an ovary or testicle, although this is not common. When a phenomenon such as those mentioned above occurs and is considered significant, normalizing this 'disturbance' is required before the osteopathy resumes work on the plications until their motility is sufficient and synchronous.

In the case of traumas or sequelae of surgery, the lateral plications must sometimes be normalized early in the sequence; however, dysfunctions of the lateral plications are much rarer than those of their thoracic and caudal counterparts.

Clinical case 2

Normalizing the lateral inflections

A man, of around 40 years of age, had undergone surgery for a kidney stone and thus had a large scar on the side of his abdomen. Although the (successful) surgery had taken place three years before and the scar had healed properly, he was feeling intense, almost constant and unsettling pain that could not be treated by his physician. The pain was quickly relieved after normalization of the lateral plication on the relevant side.

Nervous plexus

The role of the plexuses is to ensure the passage of the nervous influx from the autonomous nervous system to the viscera, which also ensures a proper vascular input for the abdominal, thoracic, and cranial cavities.

When motility dysfunctions of the two main plexuses (celiac and cardiopulmonary) are significant, they must be normalized before working on the nervous system to allow a proper distribution of the energy made available by central work to the rest of the organism, which will revitalize the cranial, thoracic, or visceral spheres without causing untimely reactions.

If the dysfunctions are not major, the plexuses will be evaluated and treated according to the reason for consultation, with a more local intervention and a focus on the dysfunctions of one or many of the structures under their jurisdiction (see the section Reasons for consultation: visceral sphere).

Neural tube folds and tentorium cerebelli

Work on the first and third cranial folds is essential to the regulation of the functioning of the autonomous nervous system. The motility of the first and third folds must be evaluated and normalized in order to regulate the orthosympathetic part of the system, whereas the motility of the first fold's lateral expansion is related to its parasympathetic part. A hindrance of the transverse movement can be caused by an incomplete movement of the first fold but also by local tensions in the tentorium cerebelli. When necessary, regulation of the membranous tensions completes the work on the longitudinal aspect of the dura mater.

Clinical case 3
Normalizing the first fold

A kinesiotherapy student, of around 20 years of age, was suffering from idiopathic colitis that lasted up to eight days and was mostly triggered by stress suffered during the exam periods. The painful episodes were progressively increasing and became out of control as they were triggered by less significant stress each time.

Eventually, normal functioning was restored to the young woman after a normalization of the first fold, because of its role in managing conscious stress, and a normalization of the celiac plexus, because of its neural and vascular influence on the colon.

To date, she has not suffered another episode in the last year. She needs to learn to effectively manage stress now that the soma has a better adaptation capacity.

Clinical case 4
Normalizing the first fold

The ability to manage stress varies from one individual to another, depending on the situation, previous emotional state, the psychocognitive schema, and the quantity and frequency of stress factors. Obviously, work on the folds does not remove all the negative consequences of stress, but it is still very useful in helping to manage accumulated stress which hinders the body's adaptation capacity and thus makes it vulnerable to the demands of everyday life.

This case concerns a 35-year-old woman who presented with secondary amenorrhea that had started after the death of her husband two years earlier. The evaluation of the first fold revealed a very severe dysfunction, and normalization of the first fold soon triggered menstruation, illustrating the importance of somatopsychic connections.

Clinical case 5
Normalizing the first fold

The autonomous nervous system is directly linked to the regulation of sleep, and, broadly, to the general state of health of an individual.

An eight-month-old baby, who had never slept more than ten minutes at a time since birth (his parents were exhausted), fell asleep on the osteopath's table and then slept for two days following treatment of the neural tube folds.

A severe restriction of the first fold is very unlikely in a child that young. After being informed of the nature of the treatment, the parents understood the source of the stress experienced by the baby. In fact, the mother had lost her previous baby in the sixth month of pregnancy; she had lived through this new pregnancy with an excessive level of stress and adrenalin that had been shared with her offspring, who had of course no means of dealing with these emotional tensions on his own.

Because of the effects on the pneumotaxic center, its superior control center, the diaphragm's movement is often freed after work on the folds if it remains hindered after work on the plications.

Clinical case 6

Normalizing the two folds

The most extreme case of respiratory function improvement occurred in a 35-year-old woman who was in a serious car accident that left her paralyzed. A tracheotomy was performed to compensate for the loss of swallowing reflex. She also needed phrenic nerve stimulation to help her breathe. At the time of the first treatment, she couldn't get by without it for more than an hour at a time. Work on the central nervous system, mostly focused on the folds and the pneumotaxic center, gave her around eight hours of autonomy after three treatments, and this increase was maintained over time.

Neurological work on the central commands of the diaphragm is of course useful in less extreme cases when the diaphragm has blockages of both the phrenic center and the cupola that resist local work.

Motility losses in a unilateral part of the first fold can help identify the effects of intense or chronic visceral dysfunctions on the nervous system.

Clinical case 7

Unilateral normalization of the first fold

Two patients aged 25 and 28, members of a family of five of which all members were suffering from hepatitis C, came to see if an osteopathic treatment could be effective. They had to decide if they were going to

start an interferon protocol since their analyses revealed an extremely high level of transaminases. The evaluation revealed very few local osteopathic dysfunctions of the liver, but the liver area of the right first fold was under a very intense blockage. Normalization of this zone, over two sessions, allowed for sufficient improvement of the blood test results, enough to delay treatment with medication.

Visceral work based on neurological engrams opens up new clinical perspectives for osteopathic intervention.

Summary

It would be very unusual to encounter a subject who is not suffering from a motility dysfunction of any of the evaluated structures involved in the three first steps of the protocol, unless the reason for consultation is very recent or regional or local only. The first three steps allow for the verification of, or ensure:

– General regulation of the autonomous nervous system;
– Decompression of the central axis, and thus of the dura mater (sometimes initiating the decompression of the lower limbs);
– Relief of the more significant dysfunctions of the cranial mechanism;
– General freedom of the diaphragm;
– General freedom of the thorax (sometimes initiating the decompression of the upper limbs);
– A general recovery effect in the visceral sphere;
– Normalization of some imprints of visceral dysfunctions on the central nervous system.

Reasons for consultation: musculoskeletal system

The motility model brings to the fore new possibilities and ways of understanding pain of the vertebral column, the pelvis, and the limbs, and parietal pain (Fig. 10.2).

Reasons for consultation: vertebral column and ribs

Pain and persisting functional disorders of the musculoskeletal system are often explained by compression phenomena of the vertebral column or limbs. As already mentioned, compressions of the vertebral column are often linked to blockages in the thoracic and caudal plications and the dura mater.

Pain is, in these cases, often spread, and it involves significant rigidity without a direct link to activity.

Costal and vertebral pains often have a visceral origin, via the tissular link or the viscerosomatic pathway. They must be distinguished from real musculoskeletal disorders. Costal and vertebral pains can also be caused by tensions of the diaphragm.

Clinical case 8

Normalizing the diaphragm and pericardial ligaments

A 30-year-old dancer was suffering from recurring pain at D4 level that was resisting treatment, even after many sessions of local manipulation carried out by various therapists over the years. At first, these sessions relieved the pain, but they had become less and less effective over time.

The evaluation showed a significant blockage of the diaphragm, which turned out to be of an emotional origin, along with a significant hindrance of the motility of the fibrous pericardium, which in turn maintained the D4 dysfunction. Several sessions were necessary in order to normalize the dysfunctions and to provide sustained relief.

In chronic situations like these, relief often occurs two or three weeks after treatment. This time period is necessary in order for the structures involved to be able to regain normal movement, which will allow for the improvement in function.

Local motility of the vertebral axis is linked to the motility movements of the notochord, the medulla oblongata, the spinal cord, and also the whole of the vertebral column. The general evaluation of the vertebral column is completed by segmental examination of the vertebrae, ribs, neural crests, spinal ganglia, and spinal nerves. Normalizing the neural crests often produces surprisingly effective results.

Clinical case 9

Segmental normalization of the nervous system

A nurse, of around 40 years of age, had been suffering from severe cervicobrachial neuralgia on the right side for a few months. Her condition was relieved by anti-inflammatory and analgesic medication. It was also partially relieved by classic osteopathic treatments that resolved everything that was seemingly local, but as the pain persisted she decided to see an osteopath who was trained in motility techniques.

During the first session, the thoracic and caudal plications were normalized, followed by the nervous system, but this was rather ineffective in relieving the pain. The second session was dedicated to lifting restrictions of these structures, giving them back a nearly complete motility; the results were still disappointing. During the third session, the osteopath tried a segmental approach for the cervicodorsal junction, normalizing the restrictions found in the spinal cord, the neural crest, the spinal ganglia, and the paravertebral (sympathetic) chain. This was very effective, and the pain soon dwindled away within a few days.

Because they allow direct intervention on the local neurological aspects, motility techniques are an invaluable clinical asset.

Motility dysfunctions of the vertebral column and ribs can be exclusively local.

Clinical case 10

Local normalizations

A patient in his fifties presented with sequelae of shingles that occurred 18 months previously. He had one scar on his skin, but it had healed properly. The shingles was inactive, but the pain persisted. The evaluation revealed a very large blockage in the rib associated with the affected region, relating to a restriction of the adjacent parietal pleura. A local treatment of the affected structures was quick and effective in relieving the pain.

Reasons for consultation: pelvis

Affections of the pelvic region are often rapidly relieved by normalization of the caudal plication, which restores motility to the sacrum and perineum, and also helps with major visceral dysfunctions of the sacrum (uterus, bladder, rectum, kidneys). This work, when a local intervention on the sacroiliac joint is necessary, can be completed by motility work on the ilium. Affections of the pelvis have various causes, not all of which can be covered here, with most of them pertaining to general osteopathic principles.

Reasons for consultation: lower limb

Pain or recurring dysfunctions in the lower limb can be the result of general compressions caused by tensions in the dura mater. These tensions must be lifted before the osteopath moves on to local motility and mobility work on the components of the lower limb.

Clinical case 11

Normalizing compressions of the lower limb

A 12-year-old child presented with a problem in the right knee. He suffered from imprecise pain when resting after playing soccer or being involved in other high-intensity physical activities. The evaluation revealed a general compression of the vertebral column and, in particular, compressions of the lower limbs, with the right limb being more affected than the left. The patient had started wearing an orthodontic appliance a few months earlier, which seemed to coincide, although with a slight delay, with the appearance of the knee pain.

Treatment consisted of relieving the tensions of the dura mater that were caused by the constraints of the orthodontic treatment. Normalization of the folds of the neural tube was also performed, along with local normalization techniques on the lower limb where necessary. Regular follow-up sessions were necessary for the duration of the orthodontic treatment to prevent relapses. Once the appliance was removed, two more sessions were dedicated to long-term relief of the structures involved in order to ensure that growth was not restricted.

The structures of the lower limb can also be affected by local motility dysfunctions.

Clinical case 12

Local normalizations

A 25-year-old young adult rugby player presented with pain in the left knee that appeared two or three months previously and which was regularly occurring after intense physical activity. Classical osteoarticular evaluation did not reveal anything conclusive, but the motility of the left tibia was extremely limited. The dysfunction seemed to have been caused by a significant impact on the tibia that happened nearly six months before emergence of the pain; it had apparently remained asymptomatic for several weeks before prompting painful symptoms. Two sessions were sufficient to deal with this rather simple problem, which was directly related to a local motility loss.

Reasons for consultation: upper limb

Pain or recurring dysfunctions in the upper limb are often affected by compressions caused by tensions in the thoracic region. These tensions must be lifted before moving on to local motility and mobility work.

Clinical case 13

Normalizing compressions of the upper limb

A retired public sector employee presented with intense pain in both hands along with swelling of the fingers, which was serious enough to prevent him from dressing. He had been diagnosed with rheumatism but medication had not been very effective. The evaluation revealed an enormous blockage of the fibrous pericardium that seemed to be the source of major compressions in both upper limbs. The treatment aimed to restore normal motility to the fibrous pericardium and to normalize the collarbone/scapula/first rib area on both sides. Results were rapid, with 50 per cent of the functions of the hand being restored after the first session. A few more sessions were necessary to end all symptoms.

Local normalizations of the upper limbs will always be more effective when the thorax (both the container and its contents) is free of dysfunctions.

The structures of the upper limb can also be affected by local motility dysfunctions.

Frequently, musculoskeletal pain in the limbs can be linked to a malfunction of the nervous system, when the latter has retained the imprint of pain (see the section Reasons for consultation: cranial field). Pain affecting the musculoskeletal system, relating to neurological imprints at the level of the sensory homunculus (parietal side of the sulcus), are referred to in Chapter 5.

Reasons for consultation: visceral sphere

Disorders relating to the visceral sphere (Fig. 10.3) have many origins. Visceral functional disorders of an osteopathic origin must be distinguished from medical, purely dietary, environmental, or lifestyle origins. Visceral dysfunctions can be linked to various traumas, caused by surgery, toxins, a physical reason, or intense or lasting emotions (see the links between the viscera and emotions in Chinese medicine). The visceral sphere is closely linked to the musculoskeletal system, which explains the frequent presence of the symptoms of visceral dysfunctions in the latter.

Clinical case 14

Normalizing surgery-related visceral dysfunctions

A 60-year-old woman presented with chronic and almost constant epigastric pain, as well as pain under the ribcage on the left side. She had had two operations for a hiatus hernia, with four or five years between the two interventions, without really having any relief from pain.

The evaluation mostly revealed motility restrictions of the esophagus and stomach, most likely caused by the pain and scars from the surgery. The primarily local intervention was preceded by the normalization of the left part of the first fold. A few sessions were necessary to significantly reduce the symptoms, and thereafter the patient attended one or two sessions a year in order to maintain the effects of the treatment, which is often necessary when the structure is affected.

Clinical case 15

Normalizing visceral dysfunctions of emotional origin

A 60-year-old newly retired businessman, who was a runner, presented with cruralgia on the left side which first occurred six months earlier. Osteopathic treatments had relieved the symptoms in the past, but had not permanently resolved the problem. The treatments had been effective for mobility dysfunctions, leaving only a motility dysfunction of the kidney that was causing a spasm of the psoas.

Normalizing the motility of the kidney and then that of the psoas were the only interventions. During the normalization, the man became aware of and verbalized an intense fear he felt a short time before the occurrence of the pain, revealing the real source of the dysfunction.

Clinical case 16

Normalizing visceral dysfunctions of emotional origin

Intense fear may cause other kinds of pain.

A 50-year-old woman, who had previously consulted the therapist for other reasons, was suffering from periarthritis of the left shoulder that appeared quickly, which seemed to coincide with an episode where she experienced intense fear. She had lost sight of her two-year-old granddaughter in a department store for several minutes, during which time she feared the worst.

Normalizing the first and second embryonic kidneys to the left and their link with the cervicodorsal junction (associated with the Dazhu [Great Shuttle]) rapidly resolved the problem, before fibrosis could emerge in the joint capsule.

Clinical case 17

Normalizing visceral dysfunctions of emotional origin

A 50-year-old woman presented with pain in the elbow (similar to epicondylitis) that was not caused by trauma or repeated movements and that had persisted for several months. Evaluation of the cervical column and the upper limbs did not reveal anything significant. However, the visceral evaluation revealed significant restrictions in the motility of the lung and the homolateral colon; as both organs are energetically linked in Chinese medicine, this principle could be useful to this clinical case. In fact, both organs are linked to the elbow via their meridians.

Normalizing the motility of the lung and the colon enabled the patient to become aware of a sad emotional event that occurred before the appearance of the pain. In this case, the patient had been close to losing her mother. As the emotion was in the past and 'inactive,' because the mother was still alive, the treatment of this visceral motility loss of emotional origin was quick and effective.

Patients do not always verbalize, or are not even always aware of the emotions behind the symptoms, and it is not the aim of osteopathy to make them aware. However, understanding and facing such situations properly are skills worth developing.

Visceral dysfunctions can also be secondary to dysfunctions of the diaphragm or disorders of the sources of innervation, or they can be linked to vascular system dysfunctions. Neural information travelling to organs and viscera comes from the superior centers of the autonomous nervous system. It passes through the brainstem toward the spinal cord, and then toward the neural crests and ganglia to reach the plexuses associated with all the organs and viscera of the body. Osteopaths must have a good knowledge of the levels of the nervous system that are connected to the various structures of the body in order to achieve satisfying clinical results.

Clinical case 18

Normalizing the plexuses

Work on the plexuses can produce results that complement local work, as in the case of a 60-year-old woman who had been suffering from effort incontinence since the menopause. Work on the celiac plexus (the bladder's innervation source), enhanced the classical osteopathic work that had already provided notable results. When evaluated a few months later, the woman stated that her symptoms were now much less of an inconvenience.

Visceral dysfunctions are sometimes part of complex clinical cases, but they are also sometimes purely local.

Clinical case 19

Local visceral normalizations

A 55-year-old patient was suffering from urinary incontinence, even after seven consecutive surgeries of the bladder and multiple perineal rehabilitation sessions that only provided a brief respite from the symptoms. An exclusively local treatment was attempted (normalizing the bladder's motility and its synchronism with the caudal plication) with very little hope of success considering the situation. The intervention was encouraging: a quick and complete

normalization of the bladder's motility was possible, to the great surprise of the osteopath. Fast-forward to a month later: the patient called to say that she would not be making any more appointments since she 'was doing 98 per cent better.'

Even with experience, it is sometimes difficult to judge the great healing capacity of the human body!

Energetic techniques are extremely useful when normalizing viscera or organs under often long-lasting dysfunctions which are undermining their vitality. These types of disorders are sometimes characterized by energy-deficiency dysfunctions that should be carefully considered by the osteopath.

Clinical case 20

Visceral energy-deficiency dysfunctions

A 55-year-old man, who was a heavy smoker, presented with episodes of lumbar blockage, which were becoming more frequent, with intense pain in the L5–S1 region which resisted classical treatments. The evaluation revealed a very intense energy-deficiency motility dysfunction of the bladder; the movement of the latter is difficult to restore. The treatment helped to reduce the intensity of the blockages but failed to eliminate them. The patient learned afterward that he was suffering from bladder cancer, which explained the persistence of the pain and the lack of success of the osteopathic treatment.

Reasons for consultation: cranial field

The possibility of working directly on the core of the cranial mechanism adds powerful tools to the osteopathic arsenal. Work on the folds of the neural tube is often the most important part of cranial work, after which classical cranial mobility work is often very effective.

Purely cranial reasons for consultation are numerous and varied (Fig. 10.4). They can include headaches and migraines, otorhinolaryngological (ORL) disorders, otitis, dizziness and vertigo, cognitive and developmental problems, etc. Considering the links between the central nervous system and the endocrine, immune, and psychoemotional systems is also essential.

When the reasons for consultation are more specific, they can be approached by the normalization of precise central nervous system zones, for example, the frontal lobe for long-term planning, ability to concentrate and social behavior, the occipital lobe for certain visual disorders, the cerebellum for equilibrium, the specific parietal lobe zone for the body schema or the left frontal parietal zone for language.

Clinical case 21

Effects of parietal pain on the central nervous system

An 80-year-old wine grower was suffering with complex regional pain syndrome (algoneurodystrophy) that had emerged after a fracture of the humerus. The fracture had not healed properly and he needed surgery to treat pseudarthrosis, but intense pain and functional losses had prevented him from having the surgery.

The treatment developed for this type of disorder was attempted, with the normalization of the first and third folds, contralateral sensory homunculus and homolateral cerebellum.

Three sessions were necessary to reduce the symptoms to a point at which surgery could take place.

In the last few years, complex regional pain syndrome has frequently been relieved using this technique.

Clinical case 22

Normalizing the hemispheres

An eight-year-old child was brought to the clinic by his parents because he was approximately two years behind at school despite being supported by a speech therapist and a special needs teacher. He had serious problems with reading and writing. The evaluation mostly revealed a significant motility deficit in the left hemisphere, which was normalized over a few sessions. The effects of treatment were progressively felt and by the age of 18 the child had caught up academically. He was supported by an osteopath (with two or three sessions a year) from the age of eight to the end of adolescence, which is also the end of the brain's period of rapid growth.

In cases such as these, the more specific and significant the motility dysfunctions are, the better the chances of helping the learning disabilities. A significant improvement after treatment of the dysfunctions

of the nervous system means that somatic elements prevailed over educational, genetic, environmental, and emotional elements, although this is of course not true for all cases.

Clinical case 23

Normalizing the hemispheres

A 12-year-old child presented with recurring sinusitis and nasal congestion that seemed to coincide with the start of an orthodontic treatment with a removable appliance. As the child was seen when energetic techniques were beginning to be developed, the initial treatment consisted of classical cranial mobility techniques for the cranial mechanism, facial bones, and reciprocal tension membranes. Toward the end of the treatment, a motility dysfunction of the frontal lobe was identified and normalized because it seemed to be mechanically linked to the symptoms for which the patient had sought treatment.

At the following session, the parents said they saw an improvement in the ORL disorders, but also a clear diminution of the child's aggressive behavior, for which the whole family had been consulting a psychologist for several months. A few more sessions were necessary to ensure lasting results until the removal of the dental appliance.

As cognitive and psychosocial development can be affected by many extrinsic and intrinsic factors, it is difficult to pinpoint precisely the impact of somatic dysfunctions and to predict the potential outcome of treatment.

Clinical case 24

Normalizing the cerebellum

A 45-year-old teacher presented with episodes of vertigo that had been coming and going for nearly three years. She is relieved by the ORL Epley maneuver applied to the semicircular canals, but the relief is only partial and short-lived.

The first treatment, which focused on the craniosacral system, sacrum, coccyx, occiput, and cranial mechanism using classical mobility techniques, produced some improvement but failed to remove all symptoms. Normalizing the cerebellum's motility over two more sessions produced more lasting results. In subsequent years, the patient came back for regular checkups, annually at first and then less frequently, even in the absence of significant discomfort. She has not experienced any further major episodes.

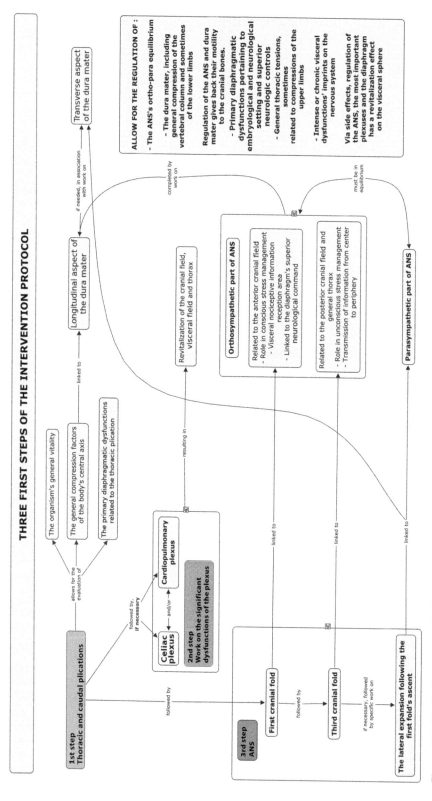

Figure 10.1. The first three steps of the intervention protocol.

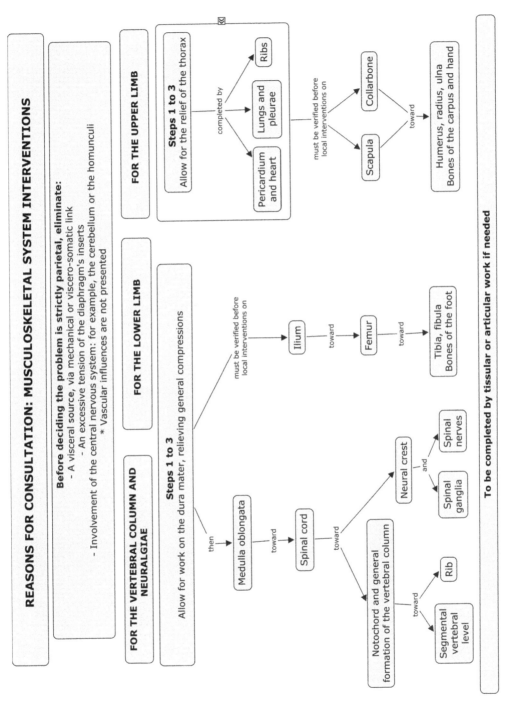

Figure 10.2. Reasons for consultation for musculoskeletal problems.

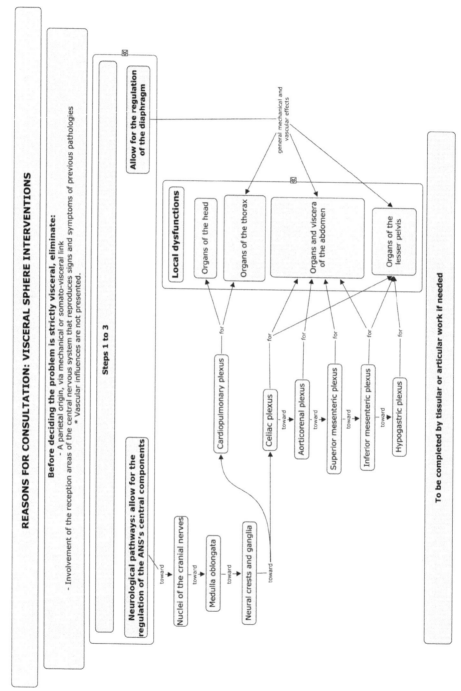

Figure 10.3. Reasons for consultation for visceral problems.

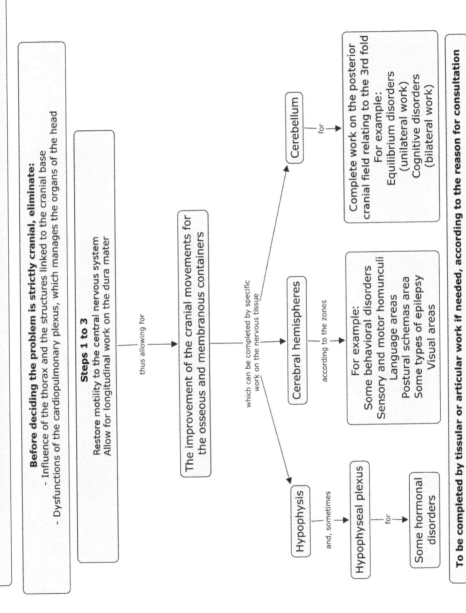

REASONS FOR CONSULTATION: CRANIAL FIELD INTERVENTIONS

Before deciding the problem is strictly cranial, eliminate:
- Influence of the thorax and the structures linked to the cranial base
- Dysfunctions of the cardiopulmonary plexus, which manages the organs of the head

Steps 1 to 3

Restore motility to the central nervous system
Allow for longitudinal work on the dura mater

thus allowing for

The improvement of the cranial movements for the osseous and membranous containers

which can be completed by specific work on the nervous tissue

Hypophysis

and, sometimes

Hypophyseal plexus

for

Some hormonal disorders

Cerebral hemispheres

according to the zones

For example:
Some behavioral disorders
Sensory and motor homunculi
Language areas
Postural schemas area
Some types of epilepsy
Visual areas

Cerebellum

for

Complete work on the posterior cranial field relating to the 3rd fold
For example:
Equilibrium disorders
(unilateral work)
Cognitive disorders
(bilateral work)

To be completed by tissular or articular work if needed, according to the reason for consultation

Figure 10.4. Reasons for consultation related to the cranial field.

Index

Note: Page number followed by f indicates figure only.